Becoming a Mother
after Thirty

Penny Blackie
with advice from Dr Janet Baldwin

Basil Blackwell

© Penny Blackie, 1986

First published 1986

Basil Blackwell Ltd
108 Cowley Road, Oxford OX4 1JF, UK

Basil Blackwell Inc.
432 Park Avenue South, Suite 1505
New York, NY 10016, USA

British Library Cataloguing in Publication Data
Blackie, Penny.
    Becoming a mother after thirty.
    1. Pregnancy in middle age — Psychological aspects
    I. Title
    306.8′743′0922   RG556.5
ISBN 0–631–14698–9
ISBN 0–631–14171–5 Pbk

c̶l̶ 308000

Library of Congress Cataloging-in-Publication Data
Blackie, Penny
    Becoming a mother after thirty.

    Bibliography: p.
    Includes index.
1. Pregnancy in middle age. 2. Pregnancy in middle age —
Psychological aspects. 3. Pregnancy in middle age — Social aspects.
I. Title. II. Title. Becoming a mother after 30.
RG556.6.B53 1986   618.2   85–15818
ISBN 0–631–14698–9
ISBN 0–631–14171–5 (pbk.)

Typeset by Oxford Publishing Services
Printed in Great Britain by Page Brothers (Norwich), Ltd

Contents

Acknowledgements

Many people helped me while I was writing this book and it has taken a long time, nearly five years on and off. Because I started working on it when my son Ben was a few months old, I had to fit it in around him. That created its own difficulties and it could have been very isolating. I thank Diane Bunyan for the enormous amount of support, practical help and criticism she offered and for her statistical expertise. Also at a very early stage I benefited from the advice and encouragement of Penelope Leach.

There were 140 contributors and without their experiences this book would never have taken shape. I thank the people who agreed to be interviewed and those who wrote, sometimes in great depth, for their openness and willingness to share what it was like for them. One of the ways of finding the contributors was by advertising and I thank *Spare Rib* magazine, *Mother and Baby* magazine, the Bristol branch of the National Childbirth Trust and the Manchester Women's Liberation Newsletter for allowing me to use their columns. Some of these people knew me when I lived in Bristol by my married name of Cleminson. I ought to point out here that Penny Cleminson and Penny Blackie are the same person.

I am very grateful to the people who read and commented on the manuscript. Doctors, midwives and nurses checked the medical detail and commented on my interpretation, for which I take full responsibility. The main medical adviser was Dr Janet Baldwin, Consultant Obstetrician at West Middlesex University Hospital, herself a first-time mother over thirty. I thank her for her hard work and good-humoured co-operation. Thanks too to

Professor Malcolm Symonds, Jane Tucker, Brenda Spencer, Dr Peter Dunn, Professor Neville Butler, Joyce Foster and Jill Rakusen.

It took a long time to reach the final stage and I greatly value the support and comments of Diane Bunyan, Vivian Sanders, Jenny Hendy, Gill Walt, Annemarie Mulholland, Jane Price, Jane Chapman and Kirsten Baker. Sue Corbett, my editor at Basil Blackwell, had the imagination to see how the first draft of the book could be developed and gave me the confidence to keep at it. Jane Katjavivi also offered very helpful advice. My thanks to them and to Stephanie Boxall.

Other people helped in practical ways: Sue Mac and Sandy Mount looked after Ben on numerous occasions; Tina Wilkinson did some of the typing and Jonathan and Joyce Bolchover kindly let me use their photocopier a lot. Clem enabled me to keep writing and rewriting by supporting me practically and emotionally. I thank him for making it possible to finish what was started. And then there is Ben, without whom. . . .

Penny Blackie
Manchester

1

Choices and Decisions: Thinking Ahead

One of the most startling changes in the birth rate in the last few years has been the increase in the number of women having their first babies after the age of 30. The last time there was such an upsurge was after the war, for obvious reasons, although it is also common for more babies to be born in times of recession. But this group of older mothers is different. For one thing, they are largely, though not entirely, white and middle class. Birth statistics in Britain are, however, collected in such a way that it is difficult to give helpful figures here. Legitimate and illegitimate live births are collected separately and since social class is judged by the *husband's* occupation, not the woman's own, it is not given for women who have babies but are not married! However, in 1982, for example, 25 per cent of mothers in social classes 1 and 2 (who were also married) had their first babies over 30 compared with 20 per cent in 1972.[1]

The average age of all mothers is rising too – from 23.9 years old in 1971 to 25.5 in 1982.[2] The graph of those figures related to social class shows that women in social classes 1 and 2 are much more likely to be older when they have their first child than women in social classes 3, 4 and 5. We are the first generation of women to have had easy access to reliable contraception, with all its drawbacks, and to free abortion. If you have an abortion in your twenties or younger, as had several of the contributors to this book, you are likely to be much more careful in future about planning meticulously when you would like to become pregnant.

Greater opportunities for higher education and professional

training have given us more rewarding jobs than our mothers might have had, jobs we are less eager to leave. Many older mothers have been busy establishing themselves in a career before thinking about parenthood, so work is a very real part of our lives, not something you do until you get married and have children. The way we organize our lives has been changing too – there is much greater flexibility about whether people live together or alone, live with one partner (a man or a woman) or with a group of people, marry or don't marry, divorce and marry again. The expectations of some women have changed enormously. They perceive their potential in a different way; they have a surer sense of themselves and what they want and have greater control over making that happen. It is this group of women who are now having babies in their thirties and forties, as part of these conscious choices.

My first child, Ben, was born when I was 35. Clem is my second husband and we had lived together for about 18 months before getting married when I became pregnant. If I had conceived in the early years of my first marriage, I would have a teenager now and I am very glad I waited. Quite apart from all the things I was able to do with such freedom, those years were an important part of my growing up and I'm pleased I didn't have to help someone else grow up at the same time. There are stores to draw on now – resilience, understanding, tolerance – and I've needed them. With some relief I gave up my job as a teacher and planned, eventually, to work part-time, perhaps at something different. I knew almost nothing about babies and didn't begin to think how it would affect my life to stay at home and look after the baby, day in and day out. I remember a friend being horrified when I told her my plans. 'But what are you going to *do* all day?' she said. I don't think I understood what she meant. I was going to cook and read, do all the things there had never been time for before. But primarily I had a vision of holding the baby close, stroking her soft skin, listening to music while I fed her – the baby was always going to be a girl. To be so completely seduced by the myth of romantic motherhood makes me feel ashamed now and I wish I had thought out some of the issues more clearly in advance. This book arose out of that realization. It sets out to examine the issues, to present information relevant to older first-time mothers and to share the experience of over 100 women and 20 or so men. The names of all the contributors and their children have been changed to preserve anonymity.

Whenever I talk about my own experiences in this book, I talk about my baby Ben. To redress the balance, where I refer to any other baby I'll assume she's a girl (and that's not because I thought Ben was going to be a girl!).

Why they waited

The contributors to this book have given many different reasons for choosing to have their first babies rather later than usual. Many of the women had been very involved in their own lives and simply hadn't got round to it before. Of those, several said that they had never had very strong feelings about babies. Those who had had a university education or lengthy professional training had been in their early or mid-twenties before they started earning. Establishing a career meant a further delay for some. A surprising number of older first-time mothers themselves had mothers who had also been over 30 when they (or older siblings) were born. Sometimes the death of a parent prompted the urge to have a baby. For some it followed on quickly after a late marriage or a remarriage.

A number of women had very little personal experience of babies. Jenny told me that the first time she had ever held a baby in her life was when she was 37 and it was her own! In retrospect she was appalled. She had treated the baby exactly like a job but, as she said, 'That was the only way I knew.' Jenny's timing was influenced by having been out of work for some months and it seemed a good way of filling what she saw as a temporary unemployment gap before she got any older.

If you are busy and don't have an overwhelming desire to have children, it can take a long time to get round to it, even if, theoretically, you are in a good position to make the decision. One of the disadvantages of efficient contraception is that you have to make a positive decision about when to *stop* using it. The very fact that you are older and more mature can make it much more difficult to decide – a totally rational approach can make you question endlessly whether you want a child to interrupt your life at all or, if you know you do, when would be a good time. Sally:

> I was conscious that I really wanted a child. It meant a working out of relationships so it was like getting married again in the sense of commitment. Not that it's necessarily any more successful a commitment but it feels like deciding again.

It was quite intimidating because after ten years of marriage you've discovered more about the wobbliness of commitments and there's much more at stake. It puts you in a peculiar position because you can't just let it happen like previous generations managed to do. There's a feeling of it being a new situation, of having to make a lot of decisions again.

Maggie and Philip were both 32 when their baby was born and they are enjoying it all enormously, much more than they expected. Maggie:

We had been married for nine years. Neither of us had been particularly baby-minded. We tended, if anything, to drop friends when they started families. We had busy careers and social lives and little contact with small children apart from during work hours. The decision to try for a baby came partly from anxiety about having been on the pill for ten years but was largely due to my increasing age and the feeling that if we didn't at least try, we may regret not having children when it would be too late for me to conceive safely.

Both partners in a couple may not feel exactly the same about having children. Chris and Robert had also been married for some time. Chris:

Ninety per cent of my motivation for deciding to have a child was the pleasure it would give Rob. He had always been fond of and empathetic with other people's children, and although he never put any pressure on me through ten years of marriage, I knew that becoming a father would be a wonderful gift to him. I felt that there was certainly space now in our lives for a child. I was 32 and it was not until earlier that year that we had our first house. Previously, financial constraints had made considering parenthood an irrelevance. So the decision was entirely mine, based on the belief that if, when past my child-bearing years, my husband grieved over not having had children, I would be full of remorse.

Other people, and perhaps an increasing number of them now, postpone having a baby for financial reasons. Rita:

We had been married for 13 years when I became pregnant for the first time at 34. We had always lived in flats or with relatives and we didn't think it was right to have a baby till we had our own house. As my husband was on low wages it took us a long time before we found a house we could afford. When we had everything we needed we decided to try for a baby. I became pregnant right away and then had twins!

Only one contributor said that she might have decided not to have a child if she had known more about how her baby's dependence would affect her life. Five babies were conceived by 'accident'. Janice spoke for most of the other women:

> I'd had ten years of adulthood, done a lot of interesting things – so I had no feeling of the world passing me by. I think I was more resilient. I had a family by choice, not because I drifted into it, and so felt and feel strongly committed to bringing them up. I feel that the years before I had children were more selfish ones. Life has been much fuller and richer since and I think being older has helped towards that. I'm possibly able to see more of the overall picture of what's happening to us just because I've lived that bit longer.

For most older women the decision to have a child is not taken lightly. A woman over 30 is likely to be more confident about what she wants and more certain about her partner than she would have been in her early twenties. The chances are that it won't be the first partner for either of you and the experience of other relationships probably makes both partners choose more carefully the kind of life they want to live together. Cathy and John had lived together for twelve years. Cathy:

> In some ways the decision to have her was connected to the decision that I didn't want to live in such a pressurized way, have such a frantic life. I've spent years of working under pressure, always to deadlines and I didn't want to do that to the same degree.
> I didn't know what I would want but it was perfectly understood between us that if we were going to have a child, it was a joint responsibility. I think at some level women choose quite carefully who they have a child with. Especially if you're over 30, you weigh up the plusses and minuses.

Very careful thinking and planning seem to precede conception for many people. Unlike some younger mothers, once you are over 30, you are often aware of all sorts of other elements in your life that are important enough to you to be built in before the baby arrives.

Fiona planned to have her baby when she did, four years after getting married:

> In my twenties I was not interested in marriage or having children. I had a full and interesting life teaching, in West Africa, then immigrant children in London. In my later twenties I began to feel I would like children of my own and even wondered about the possibilities of adopting as a single woman. However, I met Nick and we got married when I was 29, he 31. From then on I began to think more and more about babies. Nick wasn't particularly keen on the idea and in any case we needed time together as a couple before embarking on parenthood. From a practical point of view too, I was in no hurry. I wanted us to get a house in Oxford, suitable for bringing up a family – we were living in Nick's bachelor accommodation – and I wanted to learn to drive, something I had not needed in London, but felt essential here with the poor provincial bus service, to transport a child around and get to work. My job was another reason for postponing parenthood, in that I wanted to get settled in the new job and of course to earn my right to go back to the job after maternity leave. Hence there was no rush towards parenthood.
>
> I really was extraordinarily lucky in that everything turned out just as I had hoped and planned and also that everything went so well and happily.

Going it alone

You might decide to have a baby even if you know you will have to manage on your own, either because you won't get much practical help from the father or because there is no stable relationship anyway. Marian knew that her relationship with her baby's father would not last and, as she expected, when she was five months pregnant, they separated.

> I became pregnant at 36 on purpose. I had an abortion at 27, before which I had never considered the idea of having children. That concentrated my mind. I decided I definitely wanted children. I met the father of my baby in 1975 and told him from the beginning that I wanted children. He was never

keen but hope remained that he would come round to the idea. I became accidentally pregnant in 1976 and was thoroughly delighted. He was distraught. I had a miscarriage (I was silly – did some decorating, painted walls, ceilings, etc.). I was then 33 and time was running out. I made a conscious decision that I was not going to be cheated of children by time and a self-centred man and planned my course.

I carefully prepared for a life after childbirth and equipped the flat as fully as possible. There was only one thing I never had – savings. I planned when to conceive – I wanted a spring baby to grow healthy and strong during the summer. I funked it in 1978 – somehow didn't have the courage to take the plunge. By 1979 the relationship was disintegrating so much it wouldn't hold up for another year. So that, and having achieved all the preparations, decided me to get pregnant then.

I must be very fertile – I didn't try for months and months. Most people realized that 'at my age' it was a desperate act to escape childlessness and, as such, understandable. Trying to convey the intricate reasoning behind my decision to have a child and trying to justify the stand I have taken has been the most difficult thing. I feel more and more indignant that mine is a social outcast position because I am not married to the baby's father. If I'd been married no one would have castigated me for 'doing it on purpose'.

An interesting aspect of changing attitudes is the growing confidence of women to have a baby come what may. If there isn't a man in their lives more women set out to make their own arrangements and these vary from a planned one-night stand to artificial insemination, either arranged through an agency (and therefore expensive) or by self-insemination, which means finding a donor. Lesbian women who want to have a child but don't want a relationship with a man have used these methods successfully. Although it is hard to have a child on your own at any age, Marian found that being 36 helped considerably:

Before I had a baby I advocated 'going it alone'. It has been much harder than I ever thought it would be and I would never do it again. But there are lots of advantages to being over 30: assurance, confidence, the feeling that you've done a lot of the things you wanted to and the baby isn't stopping you doing them. It's *his* turn now, as it were. Also, the advantages of seeing other people's mistakes and having the benefit of a lot of knowledge about childrearing. The advantage of having developed patience and tenacity and the ability to keep going when it's very difficult. Having friends of over 20 years' standing to rely on. Having a job, maternity rights, a roof over one's head, material goodies. They're all major factors to take the edge off the difficulties.

For some women the decision to become a single parent is not taken quite so consciously or deliberately. Yvonne considered having an abortion when she became pregnant at the age of 30:

Ron and I had been living together on and off for about 13 years. At the particular time when I knew I was pregnant that was one of the off periods. It wasn't so much that the pregnancy was planned but it wasn't planned that I *wouldn't* get pregnant. For about three years beforehand we'd stopped using contraception. So, if I got pregnant that was all right and if I didn't well that was also all right. I wasn't so desperate about wanting children. If I hadn't been prepared to have him, though, I'd have been using contraception.

By the time Yvonne knew she was pregnant, Ron had gone to India where he was contemplating joining a religious community. She didn't want her pregnancy to influence his decision so waited until he had in fact decided to live there.

There was a series of exchanges of letters. I knew that we'd never got any intention of getting married so I knew he wouldn't be here seven nights a week, 52 weeks a year. It wasn't going to be that set-up. But it was really whether I was prepared to have a child on my own without the committed support of one other person to whom the child was as important as it was to me.

I wasn't at all sure that I was really strong enough to be heroic and cope. But on the other hand when I was pregnant I was very, very pleased. I don't think that terminating pregnancies is wrong but that you ought to use it as a last resort. You ought to take steps not to get pregnant and I hadn't taken those steps. I'm very good at doing what I know is the sensible thing to do, so I set out along this path but gritted my teeth.

I went down as far as the room before the operating theatre

and the guy came out and said, 'Do you really want to go through with it?' and I was going, 'No, I don't really want to go through with it but it's the sensible thing to do.' He wasn't bad. He said, 'Well, I'm not going to do it, not now, because I don't think it's the course of action you really want. I'm not saying I *won't* do it – I'm saying go away and think about it again.'

So I got wheeled back up to the ward and went to sleep and when I woke up I felt absolutely terrific. I thought thank God I backed out at the last moment. I *didn't* feel any more happy about being a single parent but I felt very relieved that I hadn't taken those steps.

So it can be a very near thing, for certainly part of Yvonne's final reasoning for going ahead and having her baby was a sense of her age and of time running out. It may be less common for a woman to have an abortion after 30 if she has ever thought of having a child at all. Yvonne was also very well aware of other factors that made it possible to contemplate being a single parent: 'I wouldn't have considered getting pregnant unless I'd got my own home, unless I'd got a job that commanded a salary. I couldn't have done it in a bed-sit on Supplementary Benefit. My age helped me make that decision. There's never a perfect time but I'd got to get the bare minimum behind me before I'd consider having a child.'

Similar practical considerations affected Marie Ely, a lesbian mother who wrote about her experiences in *Coming Late to Motherhood*:[3]

The circumstances which I had considered basic to me deciding to have a child were now, to a large extent, existing. I had always believed that parents had some responsibility to provide a secure environment for their children, and to assure them that they were wanted. My partner and I now jointly owned our own home and had some financial security behind us. Furthermore, I was optimistic that a degree of career fulfilment to date had given me some security in analysing whether I would be content to put a major part of my energy into the early years of childraising. It remained for me to decide if I really wanted to have one of my own. Throughout this time my partner wisely insisted that consideration for her should not be paramount in the decision. She said that she would support me whatever I decided, and would take on a co-parenting role if I chose to go ahead. She argued that if she had come into the relationship when I already had a child there would have been no such choice for her. The decision was therefore mine and mine alone.

Women who have had a chance to build up a job or career, the material surroundings of an equipped home, and the best possible maternity rights are more likely to be nearing or over 30 by the time they get to that stage.

Experience works for you

If you are reading this book you have probably made your decision and are thinking seriously about having a baby. You may be pregnant or already have had your baby. The experience you have had to use as a measure will probably make a considerable difference to the way you approach it all. You may well be more anxious at first than a younger woman would be because you are more used to analysing and evaluating what happens in your life and have a better idea of what could go wrong. But your maturity will certainly help you cope with the startling adjustments that have to be made once you have a tiny baby helplessly dependent on you. You will already have developed skills and resources that will help you but you'll need to be flexible enough to recognize those that get in the way. For example, if you have had a responsible and demanding job that depends on competent organization and carefully planned time, it can be difficult to let go of those efficient habits for what may be the more demanding but much less predictable job of looking after a small baby. Aleid:

> I find it really hard to adapt myself completely to his rhythm. I find it difficult that you can never finish anything. I find myself getting tense because having lived on my own so long, I could just do as I pleased. I could work all day and do everything in my own way. With him it's the complete opposite. I want to *learn* to cope with that so I do tell myself that it doesn't matter whether I do the washing up now or later or whether the house has clean floors now or next week. I really have to tell myself that because otherwise I get all frustrated because I'll want to do it and I can't. I can try and lay down my rules and schemes and what for? Just because I want the security of it? I think it's

much better to adapt to what's actually going on, to flow with it instead of trying to stick to what you want and being unhappy. It's made me a bit wiser.

Thinking Ahead

Your body

The great advantage of careful family planning is the time it gives you to ask and answer questions and prepare yourself for the birth and the time afterwards. There are lots of things you can and should think about and you will certainly get at least nine months to do it. However, there are steps you can take well beforehand to ensure that you give yourself and your baby the best possible chance of a healthy start.

Before you get pregnant If you know how your body works and look after it, you have every chance of having a normal pregnancy and birth. The risk of things going wrong does increase slightly as you get older so it is important to start from the best possible base – trying to make sure that you are healthy and avoiding the things that could increase that risk. It is worth remembering that a healthy father is important to the baby too.

The pill If you are on the pill, come off it *three months before* you try to become pregnant so that your body has a chance to get rid of the hormones and return to normal. Chapter 2 deals with conception and contraception and more detail about coming off the pill will be found on p.21.

Vitamins Recent research suggests that a lack of certain vitamins of the B group may play a role in the development of spina bifida and anencephaly. You may be short of vitamin B if you have been taking the pill or if you don't eat enough raw fruit and vegetables. A study, reported in 1980, was carried out with mothers who already had one child with a neural tube derect like spina bifida, and therefore were at greater risk. When they were planning their next pregnancy, some of the mothers took multivitamins for at least a month before trying to conceive and continued until after the second missed period. Far fewer deformed babies were born to the mothers who took the vitamins than to those who didn't. If you are not absolutely certain that you get enough of the B vitamins in your diet, it may be worth supplementing them for some weeks.

Eat healthily Your own diet will affect the health and strength of your baby even before conception. You need to be aware of the essentials of a healthy balanced diet and incorporate them into your life. This doesn't mean that you have to read books or follow charts but it does mean making sure that the food you eat is as fresh as possible and that your diet contains a good mix of protein, raw fruit and vegetables, and fibre in the form of whole grains and wholemeal bread. The more refined food is the less good it does you, so try to keep off 'junk' food or tinned and processed foods that contain artificial ingredients and hidden sugar. If you are overweight, this is a good time to try and lose some of the surplus.

Exercise Being fit will make a difference to how you feel in pregnancy and after the birth. You will be carrying a lot of extra weight around both before the baby is born and afterwards. I hadn't realized how much heavy lifting would be involved – nappy buckets and carry-cots are heavy and babies grow fast. It is a good idea to get into the habit of doing some regular exercise now. Some, like swimming, yoga or cycling can carry on through pregnancy and will be a real pleasure as a break if you keep going with them after the baby is born.

Smoking It is one of the hardest things in the world to give up smoking but there is no question that smoking damages the fetus by affecting its growth. Smokers have an increased risk of having smaller babies, premature births or even a stillbirth or neonatal death. A miscarriage is also more likely. Nature helps some women who get an aversion to cigarette smoke once they are pregnant, but you can't be sure this will happen to you. If you smoke at all, make a real effort to give it up. If you can't, get used to cutting down the number you smoke and try smoking less of each cigarette – throw it away after a few puffs. Since you absorb smoke even if you don't smoke at all, try to persuade other smokers who live with you to cut it out or down too. If you need help with giving up smoking, contact ASH (for address see p. p. 212).

Alcohol It is known that alcohol passes through the placenta and that excessive drinking can damage the fetus. A baby can be mentally retarded as a result of her mother's drinking and although it used to be thought that only heavy drinking caused damage, there is much less agreement now about what 'heavy' means. It is now thought that the risk may be quantitative and cumulative so it is worth controlling your drinking habits early. The matter might be taken out of your hands during pregnancy because many women are turned right off alcohol when they become pregnant (also tea and coffee in some cases).

If you have had an illness like hepatitis that affects the liver, it can be dangerous to drink at all. It is worth asking your GP to do a blood test to make sure the liver is normal again before you conceive. DAWN is an organization to help women who drink (address on p. 213).

Rubella Rubella (German measles) is normally a mild infection and if caught by an adult may pass completely unnoticed. Unfortunately, if you get rubella during pregnancy, the virus can pass to the fetus and may cause serious malformation. The earlier in pregnancy the illness occurs, the greater the risk to the baby. A termination of pregnancy will be offered to a woman who has rubella in the first three months of pregnancy.

About 80 per cent of women growing up in Britain are naturally protected from rubella by the time they reach adulthood. If you aren't sure whether you are immune, the best thing is to have a blood test before starting a pregnancy. Your GP will arrange this and the immunization if it proves necessary. But then it is important to avoid conception *for at least ten weeks after immunization.*

Drugs All substances that enter your body may affect the fetus. *It is therefore safest to avoid all drugs during pregnancy.* Alcohol and nicotine, of course, are drugs. If you already take a medically prescribed drug, talk to your doctor about what you should do once you become pregnant. It may be in your interest, and indirectly in the baby's interest, to continue treatment but there may be safer alternatives. If you take aspirin when you get a headache try now to find another way of dealing with the pain. It is also important to avoid 'tonics' or herbal remedies that may contain unstandardized active ingredients.

Drugs have their greatest effect on the fetus during the first three months of growth. The early weeks, when the fetus is most vulnerable, may be just the time when you are not yet certain you are pregnant. You need to be alert to the possible dangers long before you have the pregnancy confirmed.

X-rays X-rays were in use for 40 years before it was realized that they could damage a fetus. Their effect is most dangerous in the first two or three months of pregnancy when they can damage chromosomes and developing structures to cause congenital malformation. In order to avoid accidental irradiation to a woman who does not yet realize she is pregnant, X-rays involving the abdomen and pelvis are performed only within ten days of the start of a period. However, since an ovum may be developing and dividing at this time, it is wise to *avoid conception in the cycle in which the X-ray is taken.* You should always be given a protective apron to shield the pelvis from the rays.

Health and safety at work There are protective laws that lay down certain provisions particular to women at work. They cover working hours, overtime limits, meal breaks and contact with toxic substances. Time is given during working hours for antenatal checks. However, no law protects the right to have healthy children.

Pregnant women can be exposed to risks at work – risks to themselves and to the fetus. Yet no national data is collected on rates of miscarriage, stillbirth, premature birth, childhood cancer or congenital defects in relation to a woman's work during pregnancy. In fact, mortality statistics are still collected according to the husband's occupation if a woman is married, not her own.

The Health and Safety at Work Act of 1974 gives a base from which to work to improve health and safety but it is important that you know what possible risks your own job might carry. Changes in hormone levels during pregnancy make women more vulnerable to poisoning by many chemicals commonly used at work and some used at home, like household cleaners. Some chemicals are also extremely dangerous to the fetus. Threshold limits (figures that recommend maximum exposure to chemicals) are calculated according to the body-weight of the average man, so the same amount of poison might have a much greater effect on a smaller, lighter woman.

Some substances can reduce fertility or harm the fetus without affecting the woman. This means that she might not be aware of the danger; a particular problem during the first 18–60 days of pregnancy. Any substance that can harm the fetus is called a teratogen. The best-known example is thalidomide, a drug given to treat nausea during pregnancy, which caused a horrifying number of deformed babies. Following the thalidomide scandal, the Congenital Disabilities (Civil Liability) Act was passed in 1976. This made it possible for a child, born with a disability because of a breach of an employer's duty to its parent(s), to sue the employer even if a) the parent suffered no injury, b) the employer didn't know of the child's existence and c) many years had elapsed.

If you work with dangerous substances or think you might, talk to your trade union representative about it or the safety officer at work. It may be worth getting a transfer if you can or changing your job before you become pregnant rather than taking any risk.

Does your age put you at risk? While it is sensible to be aware of any possible risks if you are thinking about having your first baby over 30, don't be worried about it. When mothers over 30 are said to be a 'high risk' by some sections of the medical profession, this refers to all sorts of women, some of whom have had a long history of miscarriage, infertility or illness, while others have already had a number of children. In other words they are not really one group, all at high risk.

Preconceptual advice There are now specific clinics designed to advise people about the medical risks before embarking on a pregnancy. You should not feel that you have to seek this advice but if you have had medical problems in the past or know of instances of congenital abnormality in the family, or of a family history of illness, it might be a good idea to talk to someone before becoming pregnant. This might apply to you, for example, if you are diabetic or have chronic anemia; if you have a long history of recurrent abortion; if any members of your close family have had illnesses like tuberculosis or breast cancer. Specific checks can be made to reduce the risk. If you would like to follow this up, ask your GP to refer you.

The previous pages mention points to consider before you become pregnant. An organization that deals with that sort of forward planning and that can offer further information is

Foresight (for address see p. 213). Chapter 3 deals with pregnancy itself, chapter 4 with the birth and chapter 5 with any risks to the baby, all of them with a first-time mother over 30 in mind.

Your life

In chapter 6 I look at the first few weeks after the birth and in chapter 7 how you feel about yourself as a mother. Looking ahead, there are some other things you could usefully think about at an early stage.

There is a list of major 'life events' used by researchers and insurance companies to assess personal upheaval and stress. One of these is having a baby. Others are getting married, moving house, changing your job, coping with a bereavement. It is thought that coping with more than one of these at any one time makes life particularly difficult – a pretty obvious conclusion. Clearly you can't arrange everything that happens in your life but it might be possible to see that you don't have to move house or start a new job in the first few weeks after having a new baby, or in the last few weeks of pregnancy. If you are going to move before you have your baby, it is worth taking into consideration things like the facilities for mothers and small children in the area, whether you would be reasonably near some shops and whether it would be easy to find nurseries or childminders.

Get to know some babies All the first-time mothers who had had little or no experience of babies wished they had done something about it. They were more anxious, unsurprisingly, and tense than women who were used to small babies. When you are confronted with your very small, wriggly, seemingly fragile baby it is easy to feel clumsy and unsure of yourself. If you know other people's babies you might be able to practise putting on a nappy or doing up a babygro and you will also be more aware of some of the things that books and antenatal classes skirt round so as not to put you off! You will know that babies don't sleep all the time, that lots of them cry quite a bit, that they aren't cuddly dolls but cuddly people with needs you can't always identify but a noisy way of telling you about them. Getting to know not just your friends' babies but some in your immediate neighbourhood will give you some experience and a start in establishing the support network you will really appreciate when you have had your baby.

Sharing the chores Most of the contributors to this book live with a partner. If you live with a group of people you will probably already have a system for sharing household tasks and should be able to count on extra help when you need it. If you live on your own you will need to organize as much help as you can from your friends, especially in the weeks immediately after the birth. If you do live with a man and you both work, you will also have a way of sharing the household jobs that need to be done. But it is surprising how many women still do far more shopping, cleaning, cooking, washing and ironing than their partners. It may be worth thinking about this now and, if necessary, trying to establish a more equal division – in other words, training your man. This may not be easy if you have lived together for many years and have fallen into a way of doing things, but it is never too late to start. Babies create an extraordinary amount of extra work relative to their size and you're going to need help. If you haven't got an automatic washing machine, it is well worth saving up for one. It doesn't need to be a glistening new one — reconditioned machines at half the price often work just as well. A tumble dryer can be a real help too, although they are expensive to run.

If you are 'at home' with a new baby, whether on maternity leave or not, it is very easy to fall into the trap of thinking that because you are not 'working' you can do all the tasks that have to be done in the house. More of this later but since it can be an area of real grievance, it is worth talking with your partner very early on about how unfair these traditional roles are and how anybody who lives in a household should share the work of looking after it and yourselves.

In chapter 8 the relationship with a partner will be discussed. Chapter 9 deals with what it is like being a single parent.

Your job

A question that might exercise you just as much as whether or when to have a baby is what to do about your job after your baby is born. You may be in no doubt or you may have no choice about returning to work but whatever your own situation there are various points to think about.

The opportunities for women to work have both improved and become more constrained in the last two decades but it is still generally assumed that it will be the mother who looks after the baby and takes the main responsibility for childrearing. So if you go to work after the birth, you will probably end up doing two jobs. There are men who share childcare, even some who take on the major part of it, but it would be unrealistic to pretend that there are very many of them. The whole question of who does what is something you will discuss with your partner, if you live with a man, but in the end the responsibility might well be yours and the decision about a job will have to be a considered one.

The *image* you have of yourself as a woman may depend to some extent on your work. A job gives you not only the money to live but a clear status in the world and one you might think you feel more confident about or comfortable with than being known as a mother. If you have a job the organization of your life probably revolves around work too, so that weekends, spare time, late-night working, housework, journeys, coffee breaks, preparing meals are defined by your work in a particular way. The decison you make about your job will affect all these other areas of your life too but not half as much as the new baby will.

Chapter 10 looks at what it is like to stay at home and be a full-time mother and chapter 11 deals with women who return to work after having a baby.

Interrupting a career For people in professional or responsible, demanding jobs – women and men alike – their thirties and early forties may be the most crucial time in their working lives. You may be on an important step of the career and promotion ladder or you may be thoroughly fed up with having worked in that area for so long and be ready for a change. The mid-life crisis at work where you find yourself saying, Can I go on doing this for the next 25 or 30 years? affects both men and women and was certainly part of my decision to have a baby when I did.

An understandable concern may be that you will miss out on a stage in your working life that you look forward to or that you might not be able to cope with the job you do *and* a baby. It is worth thinking about these issues now and talking to other people who have experience that might help you. Always remember that many older first-time mothers carry on quite happily and successfully with the jobs they have, even though it is hard work. There's no reason why you shouldn't do that too. But don't expect it to be the same as it is now. You may well find that your commitment to your job or your way of thinking about it changes somewhat when you have a baby or young child to think about too. Her demands and needs, and your feelings for her, can be so strong that they affect your outlook, not to mention some of your energy.

Thinking about the practicalities Although it will be far too early to make definite plans, it is worth making local enquiries about childcare facilities (see p. 202 for the options open to you). It might also be helpful to cost out what childcare will mean to your earnings if you do go back to work. Particularly if you work part-time, or your wages are not high, you could end up paying so much for childcare that it hardly makes it worth your while, financially, to work at all. Of course, you may want to work for other reasons that compensate for that.

Outside pressure You could meet two very different kinds of pressure about working and since you may feel vulnerable when you are pregnant, it is worth being prepared for both of them. You might find yourself under pressure to go back to work even if you are fairly sure you don't want to. There may be an underlying expectation that you should be some kind of superwoman — coping equally competently with a job and a baby, when you're not sure you can manage it. That can make you feel guilty if you worry that you can't live up to it.

If you do plan to go back to work, be prepared for a fair amount of pressure from different sources. At one end is the current political pressure for women to stay at home with their children, bring them up 'properly' and relieve the employment crisis. At the other end may be your own mother or sister or neighbour who did things differently and can't see how you could do both jobs well. In between, and possibly more immediate to you is the reaction of colleagues who, for all sorts of reasons of their own, may encourage you to give up your job. All this can make you feel guilty and it is worth confronting the guilt now, recognizing it and dealing with it. *Guilt* is a special burden of women, particularly mothers, and there has never been a better time for its subtleties to be foisted upon us. We are surrounded by adverts of pretty, smiling babies and calm, pretty, organized mothers. Even when they are chasing the baby around the house trying to put a nappy on, the bottoms are always clean, the house immaculate. And both are still smiling. There is a terrible pressure to live up to the image of what a 'good mother' is reckoned to be by those powerful, manipulative outside forces. If you don't, you feel guilty. But don't be taken in by it – spot your guilty feelings now, think about them, ask whether you actually believe they are rooted in notions of substance.

What you want matters If your working life has already lasted ten years or more, then it is a very important part of you and taking account of how you feel about it matters.

- You might like your job and want to keep it.
- You might enjoy your job but wonder whether you can fit in its demands alongside those of a baby.
- You may not be happy in your job and feel you would welcome a change from it.
- You may not be all that happy in your job but feel that at least you've got one and you might not be able to get another one very easily after a gap.
- You might have absolutely no choice at all between keeping your job (or finding one) and living on Social Security.
- You may be reluctant to be financially dependent on your partner.
- You may enjoy your job but look forward to a more flexible routine and the opportunity to do other things.
- You might wonder how it will affect your self-esteem if you give up your job and become a full-time mother.

Self-interest about this decision and other things that will affect your wellbeing will make a real difference to your life with your baby. Whatever your choice it should be based on your knowledge of yourself and your reactions even though you may not be sure at this stage what you do want.

Keep your options open The maternity regulations in Britain do offer you some flexibility as long as you are eligible for them. Even if you feel fairly certain that you do not want to return to work or to the particular job you hold, you have the right to wait. It might be worth not resigning but giving yourself the freedom to see how you feel after the baby is born. More details about maternity rights are given on pp. 65–8, 207–8.

2

Controlling your Fertility: Contraception and Conception

If you are over 30 and planning to have your first baby, you have probably taken very definite steps until now *not* to have one. A small number of women become mothers after years of trying to conceive but most women will have spent that time taking a positive attitude to controlling fertility. That is a relatively new choice. Over the last 20 years the revolution in the range and reliability of contraceptive methods has made our generation the first to be able to choose the timing of our babies so confidently. That creates problems of its own – as we have seen in Chapter 1, it can make the decision about when is the right time much more difficult.

Efficient contraception also means that you can't answer the question, 'Will I be able to have children?' You may have a nagging worry that you've left it too long or that the very means of fertility control you have used may have prejudiced the chances of a pregnancy.

Can Contraception affect your Fertility?

The pill

The rate of conception after stopping the pill is the same as in those women who have never taken it. However, as has already been said, if you plan to have a baby, you should come off the pill and use a barrier method for three months before trying to become pregnant. Since the pill can reduce your absorption of vitamins B and C while you are taking it, this three months also gives you a chance to concentrate on building up these elements in your diet. There is a slightly increased risk of congenital abnormality in the babies of women who conceive within the first three months of coming off the pill or while they are still taking it.

Those three months also give you a chance to check that your periods have returned to normal after the artificial 'periods' induced by the pill. A small number of women don't resume normal periods after stopping the pill: this disappearance is called *secondary amenorrhoea*. It is not certain whether the pill itself is responsible for the loss of periods but more people believe that the pill has the effect of masking a tendency towards secondary amenorrhoea. Some women in their thirties may have started to take the pill to 'regulate' irregular and infrequent periods and carried on for contraception later. This particular form of treatment is now unpopular because of the slight risk of secondary amenorrhoea. If you had irregular periods before starting to take the pill or have experienced a delay in the return of periods during a break from taking it, it is worth coming off the pill and using an alternative means of contraception until your periods have returned. If you don't get any periods for 4–6 months, ask your doctor about it as it is usually relatively easy to sort out this problem.

The IUCD

In the 1970s there was a considerable increase in the numbers of women using intrauterine contraceptive devices (the IUCD or the coil) before having a first child. This trend was made possible by the development of a group of easily inserted devices designed to be passed through the narrow cervical canal of a woman who had not been pregnant. At the same time there was more information and awareness of the possible dangers of the pill and many women were looking for an acceptable alternative. The IUCD is an unsuitable short-term method if you are contemplating a pregnancy soon – perhaps in the next year – and should not be used while waiting for periods to return to normal after the pill.

Perhaps the greatest concern about the IUCD is *the risk of subfertility following infection* of the uterus and the Fallopian tubes. As all studies involving large numbers of users of modern contraceptive methods are still in the early stages, it is difficult to assess the extent of this problem. However, it is now generally accepted that there is an increased incidence of salpingitis (infection of the Fallopian tubes) and subsequent tubal damage in IUCD users. The risk of infection is greatest in younger women and may be related to increased exposure to infection from a large number of partners. There is also a risk of *ectopic pregnancy* occurring when an IUCD is in place – this is where the fetus becomes implanted outside the uterus, often in the Fallopian tubes. After an ectopic pregnancy, the Fallopian tube may be damaged or may have to be removed.

Planning Ahead for Pregnancy

While it is relatively simple to be able to choose *not* to have a baby, planning a pregnancy isn't always so predictable. Trying to fit a pregnancy into a vacant slot between a projected holiday and an important conference can lead to disappointment and unnecessary anxiety. Sharon, who lived with a man and his two children for a while before getting married, wondered about this:

> I went through all the mental hassle of trying to decide when would be the best time – whether to have it in the summer (thinking of things like school terms) then I decided it was all too much trouble. I'd had trouble with my periods for years so I thought I might have difficulty getting pregnant anyway and couldn't plan it as carefully as that. So I made the decision to stop using contraception when I got married and was enormously surprised that I never had another period. That was the end of it.

The very fact that you haven't been able to put your fertility to the test before may cause you to worry about whether you will be able to have a baby at all and this in turn may make you impatient. In a population of normal healthy women trying to become pregnant for the first time, the average time it takes over all ages is six months. For fertile women of 25, the average is 2–3 months.[1] There is a slow but steady reduction in the fertility of women once they are over 30 but this doesn't mean that if you are over 30 you won't conceive at all; simply that it can take longer. If you have had fertility problems or dysmenorrhoea (troublesome periods) it may take longer still, but the comment above should remind us that that isn't so for everyone.

Instead of feeling disappointed every time you get a period, you could use the waiting time to see that you are well prepared for the pregnancy when it does come. Chapter 1 outlines many of the things you can do to make life easier and healthier for you and your baby. Some of those are important before you even try to become pregnant but once you are ready to try, at least you can feel that you are doing something and not just sitting around waiting.

What to do about Delayed Conception

Possible reasons

Reduction in the frequency of ovulation Gradually the ovaries begin to function less efficiently but there is a wide variation in age and it is not usually until the late forties that they stop functioning altogether. At best there are only 12 or 13 chances of ovulation in a year, so reducing that at all reduces the chances of becoming pregnant. There is a similar but much less significant effect on male fertility with age.

Decrease in the frequency of intercourse This is probably the commonest contributor to delay in conception. If you both have busy and erratic jobs you might have fallen into a habit of making love perhaps at weekends or on specific days. If you have a very regular cycle and always ovulate on a Wednesday, say, but you tend to make love at weekends, then you may never become pregnant.

The 'best time' to conceive

Fertilization and conception is only possible for a short time in each menstrual cycle, for about three days centred on the time of ovulation. Confusion over the best time in the cycle to become pregnant is common. If your initial calculations are wrong, trying to concentrate intercourse at specific times can actually produce the opposite result. *Look at your lifestyle* and the pattern of intercourse. You need to try and match ovulation to the time of intercourse but it may not be a good idea at first to set out to do this so assiduously that you have to force yourselves to make love when you don't feel like it. Tension and strain do seem to be counterproductive in conception.

Identifying the fertile period

The fertile period is 3–4 days over the time of ovulation but the ease of pinpointing it varies from one woman to another. The methods used are based on the same information as 'natural' or 'rhythm' methods of contraception. The length of the normal menstrual cycle varies considerably from one woman to another. However, the time taken from the release of the ovum (egg) to the onset of the next menstrual period is a fairly constant 14 days. Any variation in the cycle lies in the time it takes to ripen and release the ovum. So *if your cycle is regular*, you can predict the time of ovulation.

Body temperature Recording your body temperature each day will give more precise information. The hormone progesterone produced by the ovary after ovulation causes a rise in the base body temperature of about 0.5°C over the temperature before ovulation. The fertile period extends for 1–2 days on either side of this sudden rise in temperature. There is usually a small fall in the reading just before this happens but it isn't always seen. If the information is to be reliable, you must:

1 use a fertility thermometer (ask your GP to prescribe one free on form FP10 or buy one from a big chemist);
2 take your temperature at the same time each morning while still in bed (if this isn't possible, you can calculate the difference yourself – your temperature goes up by 0.1°C every hour);
3 not eat or drink anything first.

Upheavals such as sore throat, a sleepless night or even a lie-in may cause slight variations in temperature that make the picture difficult to interpret.

Natural changes in vaginal discharge Shortly before and during ovulation the cervical mucus, usually thick and gluey, becomes thin and stringy in order to allow sperms easy passage into the womb. Many women experience an increase in vaginal discharge or an increased feeling of vaginal wetness as a result of this change. Intercourse during this time is likely to coincide with ovulation.

Observing the cervix Around the time of ovulation the cervix moves up from its usual position and after ovulation it moves down again. You can check this yourself with your finger but to do it properly you need to practise until you are aware of both positions and can recognize the change.

Other signs of fertility There are other signs that you can look out for that do not apply to all women, but may be another indicator of fertility:

1 your *breasts may be tender* around the time of ovulation and this may feel different from any heaviness or tenderness just before or during menstruation;
2 *mid-cycle spotting* affects some women and that little bit of blood may suggest ovulation;
3 a number of women have some *pain on one side or the other of the uterus* at ovulation.

Being aware of these indicators might help you pinpoint your most fertile period.

Sometimes couples are advised to *refrain from intercourse* for three days before the fertile period so the sperm count can be as high as possible. Although frequent intercourse may slightly lower the concentration of sperms, the effect is marginal. A small slip up in the arithmetic or variation in a particular cycle may result in missed opportunities. On balance this suggested time of abstinence creates as many problems as it solves.

Staying relaxed

Try not to get anxious if you don't become pregnant immediately. It is difficult to prove the correlation between tension or anxiety and slowness to conceive but it does seem to exist. It has also been suggested that women in stressful, responsible jobs that involve a good deal of tension may take longer to conceive. The very fact that doctors at subfertility clinics talk about 'holiday' and 'waiting list' pregnancies suggests that being relaxed and feeling good may have an effect on when you conceive. It may be that the harder you try and the more you think about it, the less quickly you conceive. It is worth remembering that your pregnancy and baby is to be fitted into the life you enjoy and shouldn't be intended to replace it.

When to seek help

Just as there is no 'normal' time in which you could expect to conceive, *there is no specific time* after which you should seek help if you don't. There are no rules about it and it is quite reasonable to ask for advice relatively quickly if you feel time is against you. As a guideline, there is probably little value in consulting a doctor until you have been trying to conceive for about nine months, especially if you have been aware of the factors described earlier that might help you and are fit and well. If there is an obvious stumbling block, e.g. if you have a very irregular cycle or have amenorrhoea (missed periods), it is worth taking action sooner. If you need help your *GP will refer you* to a gynaecologist or specialist *subfertility clinic* and if there is a waiting list for clinic appointments your GP may be able to initiate simple investigations him/herself. Your family planning clinic might also be able to help.

There are no absolutely agreed *estimates of subfertility* in Britain but at least 10 per cent of people have difficulty becoming pregnant and the majority of these can be helped. *Don't be reluctant to ask for advice about subfertility.* Some people feel a sense of failure that they can't achieve this very basic biological feat and might start worrying about whose 'fault' it is. It can be a very tense time, hoping each month that your period won't arrive and feeling let down or worse when it does. The tension and worry about not becoming pregnant may not just interfere with the chances of succeeding but may affect other areas of your relationships too. Friends and relatives can be the last straw with well-meaning but nosey questions about when they should start knitting. This is irritating enough if you have chosen not to have children, even temporarily, but can be very hurtful when you have no choice. So, if you have been trying to have a baby for some months and want some advice, *ask for it*. Taking some action will probably make you feel better about it too.

Investigations into and treatment for subfertility problems are available through the NHS although in some areas and for some specialized treatments, the waiting lists are long. You may be able to make out a special case if you are over 35. Most clinics are held in hospital outpatient departments, either as a specific clinic or as part of a gynaecological clinic.

For historical reasons subfertility clinics have concerned themselves more with women than men, and understanding of female fertility and how to treat any problems is more advanced than with similar problems in men. However, the causes of subfertility identified in women are only slightly more common than in men, in the proportion of about six to four – quite surprising when you think how complex our reproductive systems are. In an important minority of couples, both partners may have an identifiable difficulty. Until quite recently there was a stigma attached to going to a subfertility clinic and many men were reluctant to attend at all, let alone take part in any investigations and treatment. This may still be so for some people but things are changing and more people now go to the clinics in couples.

It is very helpful if you *and* your partner go to the subfertility clinic. It allows rapid gathering of information about your health, past medical problems, family history, sex life, and provides an opportunity for you both to be examined. It is also much better if things are explained to you together so you share equally in any projected plans and tests. The *tests* are designed to show that the vital parts of the system are all working. It must be proved that you are producing ova, that your partner's sperm production is normal and that the two meet without problems. These tests might include:

1 examining a freshly produced sample of semen under a microscope to count the sperms and see that they are swimming about actively;
2 measuring the level of progesterone in the bloodstream to demonstrate ovulation (this hormone is produced from the ovary at the site from which the ovum has been released and reaches a maximum level about a week after ovulation);
3 a blood test to measure the level of the pituitary hormones that control the activity of the ovaries;
4 checking that the Fallopian tubes are open throughout their length as fertilization takes place in the ends of the Fallopian tubes.

It is not the role of this book to go into the intricacies of the treatment of subfertility. This is a very individual matter and must be tailored to the needs of each person. The most important thing to remember is that most people attending subfertility clinics become pregnant quite independently of the help and treatment they receive there and only a minority are entirely dependent on medical intervention for success. Given that, there are drug and other treatments that might help.

It takes time Be prepared to find the process of having tests frustratingly slow. It is easy to forget that it takes time for anyone to conceive; even when your chances are normal, that chance is still only once a month. If you become impatient with yourself and the system you may actually slow down the process.

Another reason for proceeding slowly and steadily with the investigation of a couple involves the nature of the tests themselves. Although they are expensive, testing blood samples and examining semen specimens involve very little risk to the health of the couple themselves. However, further tests may involve the use of anaesthetics and minor operations, which always carry a small risk of complications. So it is better to carry out the simpler tests first. Leaping in and correcting even an obvious abnormality, such as operating on damaged Fallopian tubes, may be counter-productive if you haven't already ensured that ovum and sperm production is normal.

Calling a halt There comes a point in the treatment of some infertile couples when the doctor may call a halt, either because there is an identified problem that can't be treated in the light of present knowledge or because no abnormality can be found. It can be very difficult to accept that everything appears to be normal yet you cannot become pregnant. This can lead to a sad and destructive side to the investigation and treatment of subfertility. Gradually the motivation for attending the clinic may change from 'I'm here because I want to have a baby' to 'I have to prove that I'm capable of becoming pregnant'. Even if you are wise enough to see this happening, you could find yourself imprisoned in a system where the medical index of success is to achieve a pregnancy and the doctor will not let go until every avenue has been tried. There is a great temptation to ask a couple to return next month in the hope that there will be something new to offer or that the doctor can think of a different test to try, to mask his or her own helplessness in this situation. It is also important to bear in mind that adoption of a baby is now very difficult and that many adoption agencies won't consider a couple if they are still undergoing investigations for infertility.

AID (artificial insemination by donor) If your partner is infertile you might want to consider artificial insemination by donor. This may also seem a possible way of conceiving if you want to become pregnant but don't have a man around or don't want a relationship with a man. Ask at the subfertility clinic or ask your GP for referral for AID, but make sure you get some counselling before you take any action because this is an emotionally difficult area to deal with on your own.

If you are on your own or lesbian you might find it easier to work through the British Pregnancy Advisory Service (see p. p.212). Or you could do it yourself by finding your own donor. A pamphlet called *Self-Insemination* (see p. 216) tells you how to set about it. There is an informative account of a lesbian couple who did just this in *Coming to Motherhood* (see p. 216) which shows how much difference it makes to have the support of someone close to you while you are going through the process. The BPAS is now screening all donors for AIDS as there are a few cases of women who have contracted the disease through artificial insemination.

In vitro fertilization If you cannot become pregnant you could consider *in vitro* fertilization. This may be especially appropriate if there is an identified reason for not being able to conceive – severely damaged or absent Fallopian tubes, perhaps, or a subfertile partner. The process, which involves fertilizing an ovum outside the uterus and then replacing it, has received a great deal of publicity and is a solution to some people's infertility problems. It is not, however, always successful and there can be long waiting lists for NHS treatment. Private treatment tends to be very expensive.

Reassessing Contraceptive Methods

When you stop using contraception in order to try and become pregnant, you might breathe a sign of relief and think, well at least I don't have to concern myself with *that* for another year or so. That may be true, but that very space of time might afford a good opportunity to think about what method will suit you best after you have your baby. I remember after I had mine being quite startled when the registrar came to discuss my future contraception before I left the hospital. I hadn't thought about it at all and at that time it was the last thing I wanted to think about.

However, if you are over 30, and especially if you are over 35, you do have to think about contraception. Breastfeeding does seem to be an effective method of birth control in some Third World countries where the baby can feed on demand whenever she wants, perhaps every hour or two. In industrialized countries where we don't carry our babies with us in the same way and where our diet is substantially different, *breastfeeding does not normally provide reliable protection*. What is known as *ecological breastfeeding* is believed to protect but certain stringent conditions must be fulfilled (to do with frequency of sucking, diet and so on). For further details of how this works contact the Natural Family Planning Centre (for addresses see p. 213). Having a choice about whether or when to have a second child could make a real difference to you. If you plan a two- or three-year gap, an accident that reduces that to a year could make life more difficult for you.

The best method

It is not easy to decide on the best method of contraception. There have been many studies, particularly on the effects of the pill, and some of these have led to scares approaching panic. What has clearly emerged from all the research is that there is *no method of contraception that is entirely safe* on both the counts of avoiding unwanted pregnancy and of risk to the health of the woman. Perhaps more successful methods would have been developed more quickly if men had babies too. Taking a long-term view, we simply don't know enough. All the studies are still in relatively early stages: the evidence so far can prove that the pill or the IUCD *do* have certain effects but cannot yet prove that they do not.

Like many other women you may wish to use a method that you can control yourself. There is a noticeable increase in the popularity of the diaphragm and other barrier methods. The Tietze Report, which compared death rates associated with contraception, recommended that *for women over 35, careful use of the diaphraghm is the safest method of contraception in terms of mortality*, with early abortion as a back-up.

Contraceptive Choices for Women over 30

You will have your own views about the method that suits you. However, you might like to know about any risks known to be related to age and also about some of the more recent developments so you can make an informed choice if you want to change or reconsider.

The combined pill (containing oestrogen and progestogen)

It has been known for some time that the combined pill has a systemic effect – it affects not only the ovaries but the whole body. The long-term implications of that are not yet known. Two extensive surveys carried out in 1974 and 1977 by the Royal College of General Practitioners showed that certain women taking the pill were more likely to suffer from heart disease and raised blood pressure than women who did not take the pill. By then it was already known that the pill increased the probability for a small number of women of abnormal blood clotting, leading to deep-vein thrombosis and the danger of pulmonary embolus, the lodging of detached blood clots in the lungs.

Risks The risk of *thrombo-embolism* does not appear to be associated with age but it makes the pill unsuitable for any woman with a history of abnormal blood clotting. The most recent studies on specific risk factors suggest that the extent to which smoking outweighs other risks like obesity and age alone has been underestimated. The women particularly at risk of *heart disease* and *raised blood pressure* are smokers over 35. If you do not smoke and are not overweight you could go on taking the pill until your early forties.

Worrying publicity In October 1983 two articles were published in *The Lancet* which were taken up by the national press and caused a great deal of anxiety amongst women who take the pill. They linked the pill with breast and cervical cancer. As a direct result of this publicity many women stopped taking the pill altogether. Without going into too much detail, these two articles are a good example of how little information is really available, but how dramatic publicity can create real fear.

The other side of the coin, which seldom gets a mention, is that the pill is probably protective against cancer of the ovary and the endometrium and that benign breast disease is less common amongst pill-users.

The mini-pill (progestogen only, the low-dose pill)

The progestogen-only pill is often offered as an alternative to women who have been advised to stop taking the combined pill, or to breastfeeding mothers for whom the combined pill is not suitable. It is not yet clear whether the taking of the mini-pill leads to increased risks of complications as women get older, as the studies into this aspect are still at an early stage.

There are some disadvantages to the mini-pill. It is not quite as reliable as the combined pill and to be effective it must be taken at the same time each day. If you take it as much as three hours late you are advised to use additional contraception for the next fortnight. Some women experience irregular bleeding on this pill. If a woman does become pregnant while taking the progestogen-only pill it is more likely, as with the IUCD, that the pregnancy may be ectopic, i.e. the fetus becoming implanted outside the womb.

This pill is frequently recommended for breastfeeding mothers. Some of the hormone does pass from the mother to the baby in the milk and it is not known what long-term effect this may have on the baby. It has been suggested that some babies who are breastfed by women taking the mini-pill are more likely to be 'cranky' or unsettled. It has also been suggested that the constant presence of progestogens may increase the incidence of depression. Some women with postnatal depression notice an immediate improvement when they stop taking this pill. Another effect for some women is a dryness in the vagina which leads to discomfort during intercourse.

The morning-after pill

The morning-after pill is a recent development and it is not recommended that it be used on a regular basis. If you have intercourse unexpectedly and are unprotected or are using a barrier method that fails, it is possible to take this pill between 6 and 72 hours after intercourse to try and avert pregnancy. It uses a large dose of combined oestrogen and progestogen which is repeated 12 hours later. It probably justifies its reputation as an insurance policy as long as you don't expect to use it often. It can be very useful if you are using a barrier method, for example, which fails – a fairly rare occurrence. However, if it doesn't work it may be worth considering a termination because there may be a risk of malformation in a baby developing after this pill has been taken. There is also a slight risk of ectopic pregnancy with this pill.

The IUCD is also good post-coital contraception and is effective if inserted within five days of intercourse (and, of course, once in, could be an acceptable long-term measure).

The IUCD

There are no grounds for thinking that a woman in her thirties is at any greater disadvantage using an IUCD. Indeed, many of the studies highlighting the risks of this method indicate that older women may have fewer problems than those in their teens. The most common effects are heavier periods, more painful periods or periods that last longer. If you already have heavy periods or are at all anemic, the IUCD will probably not suit you.

Depo-Provera

The idea of a long-acting injection that will protect against pregnancy for months without the need to remember to take tablets or use a mechanical device is an attractive one in theory. However, some people have reservations about the long-term safety of Depo-Provera. It has been widely used in Third World countries despite suggested links with breast cancer, infertility and amenorrhoea. In Britain there has been a campaign against Depo-Provera, particularly against giving it to women without their knowledge or informed consent. It may not be a good idea to use it immediately after giving birth, which is sometimes suggested to new mothers while they are still in hospital. There are some recognized side-effects but not enough is yet known about its long-term effects.

Barrier methods

If you are in your thirties or forties and became sexually active in the era of the pill, the idea of using condoms or diaphragms can seem distasteful. But these methods are gaining in popularity.

Although they have never been considered as reliable as the pill or the IUCD, the failure is usually because of the way they are used. Older women tend to be more at ease with their own bodies and highly motivated about controlling fertility, so they use barrier methods effectively.

You could try out *a number of methods* and then combine those that suit you. Don't be put off by the instructions that come with many devices – some of them are very cautious indeed. Much depends on how important it is to you to achieve 100 per cent reliability or whether you might be prepared to take a slight risk, given that many women over 30 are not quite so fertile anyway. Furthermore, many of the recommendations about how to use barrier methods owe more to tradition than to scientific evidence. Some of the 'rules' are very important, but there are so many of them, often treated as equally important, that it can be hard to know where to concentrate your greatest effort.

If you want to know more about this, the *British Journal of Sexual Medicine* has published recommendations about which of the instructions for barrier methods are really relevant.[2]

The diaphragm There are two kinds of diaphragm available – the flat and the coil spring, although you are likely to be offered only one of them at your family planning clinic. If you find your diaphragm uncomfortable after the birth of your baby, as some women do, ask for the other kind which might fit you better.

Cervical cap There are three kinds of cervical cap to try, so if you like the idea of this method, you should be able to find one that suits you.

Spermicides There are many different kinds of spermicides and various ways to administer them. In Britain it is usual to suggest only using spermicides together with another method. However, in some countries, notably France, they are often used on their own successfully. Like the condom, spermicides can help to prevent infection.

Vaginal ring This is a new device still at trial stage but it is going into production and should be available in 1986. It is a small ring of silastic rubber, 2 inches in diameter and as thick as a pencil. It is placed in the vagina and stays there all the time. By releasing a small amount of progestogen at a slow and constant rate, the ring works to thicken the mucus of the cervix so the sperms can't get through. It doesn't affect ovulation or the rest of the body and needs to be changed only every three months.

Vaginal sponge A small sponge impregnated with spermicide can be placed in the vagina 24 hours before intercourse and left there for at least 6 hours afterwards. It is already quite popular in the USA and is gradually becoming available in Britain. It is not quite as effective as the cap or diaphragm.

Condoms Condoms are still the most widely used method of birth control in Britain. Some of the women who want complete control over their own fertility feel that the main disadvantage of this form of contraception is that it puts the control firmly and literally in the hands of men, but women can put them on too. Condoms are a much more positive proof of contraception than, say, the pill.

Advantages of barrier methods The methods themselves do not interfere with the normal working of the body and therefore have no adverse effect on future fertility. A small number of people who have had difficulty conceiving because antibodies have formed in the woman's body against her partner's sperms, attacking and destroying them in the vagina and the cervix, have found that using a barrier method may allow the system to return to normal. Barrier methods also protect against venereal infection and may reduce the danger of developing cervical cancer in later years. Such methods also have a place in allowing a breathing space for the body to return to normal between coming off the pill and trying to become pregnant again.

Natural family planning

You may find that natural methods suit you best. As women get to know more about how their bodies work and become more conscious of controlling all aspects of their health in so far as they can, these methods have gained in popularity. The physiological markers of ovulation time are used to indicate the fertile time of the cycle when intercourse should be avoided. You use a combination of counting days, taking your temperature, examining vaginal mucus, measuring vaginal fluid and observing the cervix to predict when ovulation occurs. There are also more minor signs of fertility, not necessarily experienced by *all* women, such as the tenderness of your breasts, mid-cycle spotting and pain felt around the time of ovulation. This method uses exactly the same information, in reverse, as you use to plan the right time to try and conceive when you *do* want to have a baby (see p. 25).

Sterilization

Sterilization is sometimes seen as a very convenient method of contraception for an older woman who does not want to have any more children. If you and your partner decide that one pregnancy and one baby is all you wish to have and that sterilization for one of you is your choice of future contraception, that choice should be yours alone.

However, you would be well advised to wait until your baby is at least two months old before committing yourself to the operation. This also applies if your partner is considering vasectomy. For a woman, there is a slightly higher risk that the operation will be unsuccessful if it is done soon after the birth, before the uterus and the Fallopian tubes have involuted to their pre-pregnancy state. More importantly, the time immediately after the birth (or after a termination of pregnancy) is not a good time psychologically to make a long-term decision about fertility. There is more chance of suffering regret, postnatal depression or of wanting the operation reversed if the decision is made before at least a couple of months have elapsed.

3

Pregnancy

You will probably have read or be planning to read other books on pregnancy and childbirth. One thing older mothers have in common apart from their age tends to be an absorbing interest in what is happening to them and a helpful urge to know all about it. Knowing what the stages are and what is likely to happen to your body and the fetus inside you, is a very reassuring way of dealing with such a new experience. It is not the purpose of this book to describe all aspects of pregnancy, but rather to point to those factors of special interest to a woman over thirty having her first baby. The list of books on p. 215 contains suggestions of other books that give a much fuller general picture.

The information given in this chapter is intended to dispel anxiety rather than create it. A normally healthy woman over the age of 30 can expect to have a normally healthy pregnancy. However, some of the problems which may arise to complicate a pregnancy become more frequent as the age of the mother rises over 30, and especially if it is to be her first baby. It is your right to know what these problems are even if they are unlikely to happen to you. To be aware of your body and alert to any possible difficulties makes it easier to cope with problems should you be unlucky enough to have any.

In his book *Pregnancy*, Gordon Bourne, then Consultant Obstetrician at St Bartholomew's Hospital, London, says, 'Pregnancy and labour presents certain risks to the elderly primigravida, but with proper antenatal care and good supervision during labour, these are negligible. Indeed, maternal age should never be used as a deterrent to establishing a pregnancy.'[1]

What is an 'elderly primigravida'?

A primigravida is the term used to describe any woman who is pregnant for the first time. You might come across the word 'primipara' too, which also means a first-time mother. The medical profession has tended to call any 'primigravidae' over 35, or in some centres 30, 'elderly' as a sort of shorthand to indicate the slightly higher risks women over that age may run in pregnancy. You may feel insulted to be referred to in this way and fortunately some doctors are beginning to realize this and use the phrase 'maternal age' instead when assessing risk factors. Being singled out by your age alone can make you feel unnecessarily anxious so it is important to remember that most women over 30 have a normal pregnancy and delivery.

Being pregnant

Once you are actually pregnant, you might feel quite different very quickly. A number of women know they are pregnant after a very short time, long before the pregnancy can be confirmed, simply because their bodies feel different. For example, your breasts might feel especially sensitive. You will probably feel excited and delighted but don't be surprised if you also feel confused, overwhelmed and astonishingly tired. Fortunately the tiredness wears off after a few weeks and so should any nausea you might have. So-called 'morning sickness' *can* go on all day and the nausea, on top of the tiredness, can make early pregnancy a difficult time. Many women could do with time off work at the beginning rather than at the end of their pregnancies. If you have to work and it is a busy time, try to pace yourself so that you get as much rest as possible. Go to bed early and eat healthily. But don't worry if you can't eat much. I survived on a diet of toast and marmite (which was all I could face) for three months. Frequent small meals often help to allay nausea.

A few women feel uncomfortable and lumpy and don't enjoy being pregnant but far more do. Once the first 12–14 weeks are over, you should feel well and energetic and it is often a real pleasure to be pregnant. As Gill said: 'It's the first time in my life I haven't been unhappy about my body simply because for once nobody cared what weight I was. I was the one with the lovely big belly.' You might not feel quite so much at ease with the number of people who seem to think that because you have a baby inside your big belly, it's OK for them to stroke it. People do treat you differently when you're pregnant, so be prepared for that. You will probably enjoy the concern and the help and the cherishing some of the time but it can be a bit much if colleagues and other people you have to deal with (mostly men) assume that as your body gets larger, your brain gets smaller.

Attitudes of the medical profession

The way your GP or, later, a hospital doctor reacts to your age will depend on that person and perhaps the prevailing attitudes of the area or hospital. There does seem to be shift in attitude since so many women in their thirties started having first babies. Because it is less unusual, fewer doctors comment on age. When I expressed some anxiety about being 34 on my first visit to the hospital, the doctor said, 'What are you worried about? This is a perfectly normal pregnancy.' That was reassuring but I am also quite certain that a special note was made of my age. Most of the contributors to this book were pleasantly surprised at how little fuss was made about their age.

All the same, be prepared for the odd careless remark which might be hurtful, the more so because it is made at a time when you might be feeling vulnerable anyway. Liz, who was 37 when she became pregnant, was made to feel that she was contravening the rules: 'Our GP made a number of remarks about my age. It's not good because it can't actually make any difference then. There you are, you're pregnant, so what use is it saying things like "at your age". It makes the check-ups rather unpleasant. I can see why people stop going to them.'

Care during Pregnancy

If you are healthy, understand how your body works and look after it you are likely to have a happy and trouble-free pregnancy whatever your age. It is very important to take good care of yourself during pregnancy for your own sake and the baby's sake, since there are so many ways of accidentally affecting the outcome of the pregnancy. It has been shown that many risks to the fetus are related to social and economic disadvantage, poor education, inadequate antenatal care and extreme youth. The higher the social class, it seems, the lower the risk to mother and baby.[2] Age here is a positive advantage in that as an older woman you are likely to be both more knowledgeable and more highly motivated about looking after yourself. If you have not yet read the section in chapter 1 about looking after yourself and avoiding things that could be harmful (on pp. 11–15), read it now. All the points about general health and nutrition, exercise, vitamins, smoking, alcohol, drugs, X-rays and dangers at work apply just as much, if not more, now that you are pregnant.

Regular antenatal care will offer one way of checking that the pregnancy is progressing normally. Routine tests of urine, weight gain, blood pressure and blood tests will reveal any problems at an early stage and since some things that can go wrong (like raised blood pressure) don't have any identifiable symptoms, it is much the safest thing to have these checks regularly. There is legal provision for all women to have paid leave from work to attend antenatal clinics although this may not apply to you if you work part-time (i.e. less than 16 hours a week). The antenatal care that will be offered to you will depend on your decision about where to have the baby, so that is something you need to think about early on.

Options open to you about where to give birth

At home There has been a very strong move towards hospitalization for all births in Britain, so very few babies are born at home – about 1 per cent. You would probably be discouraged from having your baby at home if you are over 30 and it is your first baby – both these factors are believed to carry a greater risk. However, some women feel very strongly that they want to give birth in their own homes and have been able to arrange it.

Annie found it surprisingly easy. She had had four miscarriages and didn't want to go back into hospital to have her baby. The baby's father is a doctor and they set about getting a home confinement. She was 33 so suspected that they would have to be very well prepared, particularly in view of her past miscarriages. By asking around they found a GP who was willing to take her on. She and Don went together to the hospital for her 16-week check-up, armed with a letter from her GP and a pile of statistics; expecting to have to fight to get agreement to a home confinement. Much to their surprise, the obstetrician agreed. 'That's up to you,' he said. And that was it.

You have a right to a home confinement but it isn't always so easy to arrange and the dealings can be unpleasant. Make sure you are single-minded about it, stay calm and pleasant and firm and do your homework. The Society to Support Home Confinements (address on p. 214) offers very helpful advice to any woman wanting to pursue a home birth, giving information about your rights and the draft of a letter you can write.

If you are booked to have a home confinement, all your antenatal care will be carried out by the midwife who has been assigned to deliver you, and your GP, if one has agreed to the procedure. This should mean that you see the same people each time and have complete continuity of care.

GP unit If you have a bed in a GP unit in a hospital, your GP will be responsible for your antenatal care and will come to the hospital when you are in labour. You will probably also be checked by your community midwife antenatally and she will deliver you in hospital. If there are complications, other medical staff might be called in. Whether or not a GP unit will accept a woman over 30 (with a slightly greater risk of possible complications) might depend on whether the unit is an integral part of the hospital, with other help easily available, or rather more isolated.

Domino unit Some hospitals have a 'domino' unit (which stands for domiciliary in-and-out) where you can be admitted to hospital just for the birth itself, accompanied by your own midwife who will stay with you for the birth. Normally you can go home six hours after the birth and the same midwife will care for you afterwards, offering complete continuity of care. This may be possible in a GP unit or a consultant unit in the hospital – the difference is in the emphasis on a short stay.

In hospital If you opt for a hospital delivery (and most women do) you will go to the maternity ward of a general hospital or a specialist maternity hospital, depending on where you live and the facilities available. You will see the hospital staff at least three times during your pregnancy, seeing your own GP and midwife in between. You should be offered the opportunity to look around the delivery rooms where you will give birth. In hospital you are much less likely to see the same doctor or midwife each time and it is quite possible that, although you are 'under' a consultant obstetrician, you will never meet him or her. You should have some choice of which hospital you go to. *The Good Birth Guide* by Sheila Kitzinger gives details of the relative reputations of many hospitals to help you make your choice.

Antenatal visits

It is important that you keep your antenatal appointments but it is also easy to see why many women don't value their visits. There may be an inefficient appointments system which keeps you waiting for longer than seems necessary and, when you are seen by the medical and nursing staff, you can feel as if you are being treated as part of a production line where things are done *to* you. As a woman of some experience, used to operating competently in the world on your own behalf, you may well find antenatal clinics particularly irritating. If you are not used to being talked down to in your everyday life, it is difficult to take this from doctors or medical students who may be much younger than you are. Instead of being treated as a prospective mother looking forward to having your baby, you find yourself classified as a 'patient' who has an illness – pregnancy.

It is well worth expecting some of these irksome aspects of antenatal care and reminding yourself at every stage of your dealings with doctors that they are just people. They certainly have skills you may need but they also work in a powerfully hierarchical atmosphere which might not always encourage patience and tact. A chance or clumsy remark can haunt you. Pauline:

I had three appointments at the hospital before the baby was born. At the first one (the appointment was for 9.15 a.m. and I finally left the hospital at 12.15) I was seen by a doctor and two medical students. I was 34 weeks at this stage. The doctor asked the students what was peculiar about me and they said my age. He agreed and asked them what they should be looking out for. They replied 'blood pressure' and a couple of other things I knew about and then one said they would induce me at term. I asked the doctor why and he said because there was a higher chance the baby would 'just die in the night' in older mothers. I never forgot that and in the last week of my pregnancy became quite neurotic about it, especially when subsequent doctors disagreed and when, on the day the baby was due, they gave me an appointment for two weeks' time!

This account is not included as a horror story. It illustrates very well certain aspects of antenatal care that you might watch out for.

- You frequently have to *wait a long time for your appointment*. This is one of the strongest complaints women have about antenatal clinics. It can seem like an assumption that pregnant women don't have much else to do and can be kept waiting, sometimes for hours, for what might turn out to be a few minutes of examination and questions. This can be worse with subsequent pregnancies, if you have no alternative to taking a toddler with you too, which does happen to some women. To avoid getting angry and upset (and inadvertently raising your blood pressure!) arrive on time for your appointment, expect quite a wait and take something to do. You are much less likely to get annoyed if you can use the time to read your own book or write a letter.
- There may be *students* present at your antenatal checks or indeed, later, during your labour. You should be asked whether you mind about this and if you do, say so. You do not have to agree to take part in teaching. On the other hand, students can provide a less authoritarian access to more information if you get a chance to talk to them.
- Some doctors, as appeared to be the case with Pauline, talk *about the woman* as if she is not there. There are few things so irritating to a woman who is used to controlling her own life, as being treated as if it is just her body that is giving birth and that *she* doesn't matter.
- When Pauline asked a question, the doctor gave what seemed to her a *patronizing* and unsatisfactory answer – that the baby might 'just die in the night'. This is a very sweeping statement without further explanation and it isn't surprising that she was alarmed and upset.

Getting the information

There are various things you can do to make certain that you do get the information you want. Apart from reading and going to antenatal classes (see p. 60) you need information that is particular to *you* and *your* pregnancy. At your first antenatal check you may be given a *co-operation card* which records all sorts of information about your pregnancy. Get someone to explain the symbols to you (or look it up in one of the books listed on p. 215).

Before your next check-up write down the questions you want to ask and make a note of any worries so that you don't forget what they are when it is eventually your turn. Having asked a question, it is important to listen to the reply and come back on anything you are not sure about. Sometimes, if you are given a lot of information at once, you latch on to one bit and don't fully 'hear' the rest. Keep asking until you have received a satisfactory answer but if one person is a bit cool, brusque or off-putting, try another. Once you find a GP, midwife, hospital doctor with whom you have a rapport and who you feel takes you seriously, ask to see that person on subsequent visits. In hospital this may not always be possible, but it is worth asking. Try to meet and talk to your community midwife before the baby is born. You will see her regularly in the first fortnight after the birth so it is particularly helpful to get to know her in advance.

On all sorts of matters affecting pregnancy and childbirth, there is *no consensus*. Doctors will have different ideas and different ways of dealing with the same situation. If you have a fair amount of information at your fingertips, at least you will know what questions to ask to find out what you need to know.

Antenatal Tests

Like any pregnant woman you will be offered a number of routine antenatal tests:

1 a blood count to detect anemia;
2 identification of blood group;
3 a test to detect sexually transmitted disease;
4 a check to ensure immunity from rubella (German measles). If you are not immune and think you have been in contact with disease in the first four months of pregnancy you can have further tests to show whether you, and hence the fetus, have been infected. You can then be offered a termination of pregnancy if you wish. If you are not immune, immunization can be given in the first few days after delivery to offer protection for the next pregnancy;
5 a urine check for the presence of infection or kidney disease.

In many centres other more specialized tests may be available.

Some of these are particularly useful in helping to combat the disadvantages faced by older women, especially those approaching 40. It is an extraordinary medical advance that a diagnosis of certain defects can be made before the baby is born, through techniques like ultrasound scanning and amniocentesis. More sophisticated tests, some of which involve identifying defects from the blood of the mother, are also being developed. Because the vast majority of babies are born quite normal, the specialized tests are usually only carried out on selected women considered to be at risk.

However, some women are not happy about some of these 'advances', seeing the whole issue of technological intervention as a moral issue about how far it is reasonable to go in the prevention of possible problems. If you feel like that it will be up to you to decide what is appropriate for you and at what stage of any suggested tests you might opt out.

Alpha-fetoprotein

Alpha-fetoprotein is a chemical produced by the developing fetus. It is present in high concentrations in the amniotic fluid and to a lesser degree in the mother's blood. The reason for its production by the baby is unknown but it is well-proven that the level rises dramatically in the presence of certain abnormalities in the baby. Neural tube defects, particularly anencephaly (where the brain is not developed) and spina bifida produce this change, as do a number of rarer conditions. The level of the chemical is closely related to the age of the pregnancy so if there is doubt about dates and the length of the pregnancy, the test cannot be interpreted. In the presence of high levels in the blood test, an amniocentesis is usually performed (see p. 48) to confirm the results. Termination of the pregnancy would be offered if a problem was identified. A new and more reliable test is under investigation.

Testing for AFP is routine practice in some hospitals but if this is so, you should be told about it. You may not want to know whether there is a fetal abnormality and would be able to decline the test.

Ultrasound

How it works Ultrasound is a technique that was developed by industry and successfully adapted for use in medicine. It has been in use in obstetrics since the early 1960s and the range of application and availability of the test is increasing. It works by sending out very short pulses of high-frequency sound energy into the body, listening for the 'echoes' to return and converting these patterns into a picture form, which can be shown up on a screen like a television set.

The gel or oil which is spread on the abdomen of the pregnant woman helps to conduct the sound beam. Each time the energy passes a junction between two different substances, some of the sound is reflected back and helps to draw a plan of the body structures. The sound waves pass particularly easily through liquid allowing a good view of the fetus floating in the amniotic fluid. A full bladder also helps to improve the picture by lifting the uterus up out of the pelvis where it is hidden from the ultrasound beam. The evidence available shows that it does not cause significant changes to the chromosomes in the cell nuclei as X-rays do. It has generally been considered to be non-invasive and safe but a recent American study raised questions about a higher incidence of learning difficulties (specifically dyslexia) in babies who had been exposed to ultrasound *in utero*.[3] Subsequently the Royal College of Obstetricians and Gynaecologists set up a working party to look at the safety of ultrasound. This report confirms the weight of evidence of the safety of the technique, 'however, pregnant women should not be persuaded into the examination against their wishes'.[4] There is a good deal of controversy about the use of ultrasound scanning on a *routine* basis which will continue until further studies are carried out.

Uses There are some specific uses for ultrasound that can be very helpful in increasing the safety of a pregnancy:

- It gives an accurate assessment of gestational age, i.e. how many weeks on the pregnancy is. This is particularly important if you are uncertain of your menstrual dates, have irregular cycles or have recently taken the contraceptive pill. This information is very important if pregnancy complications develop and the baby does not grow well in the uterus, perhaps leading to the advising of induction of labour.
- It can help diagnose miscarriage, e.g. if there has been vaginal bleeding, a scan will show whether there is an embryo, and whether the pregnancy is viable.

- It can help diagnose an ectopic pregnancy. This is where the fetus starts developing somewhere other than in the uterus, e.g. in a Fallopian tube.
- It can diagnose *placenta praevia*. In these cases the placenta has implanted in the wall of the uterus close to or covering the inside of the cervix instead of its normal position in the upper two-thirds of the uterus (see p. 59).
- It can diagnose multiple pregnancy.
- It will reveal certain fetal abnormalities, e.g. anencephaly, hydrocephaly and spina bifida.
- It is especially valuable preceding an amniocentesis.
- It is possible to use ultrasound to aid in the diagnosis of congenital defects like heart and kidney abnormalities, although this may require sophisticated high-resolution machines.

Ultrasound is a painless procedure that many women find very exciting:

> I found this a very rewarding experience as for the first time in my pregnancy the baby became a reality. Not having felt movements (it was too early), to see my baby moving about was indescribable. Combine this with the knowledge that it seemed to have all the necessary limbs and appeared, as far as was possible to tell, quite normal, it was a very reassuring thing. The physical side was very relaxing as the staff talked to me through the process and translated the projection on the screen so that I could understand what was happening. There was no discomfort. I regretted the fact that although my husband accompanied me to the hospital, he was not invited to see the scan. I think he would have found it as amazing as I did.

Amniocentesis

The purpose of amniocentesis is to withdraw some amniotic fluid surrounding the fetus, separate the fetal cells it contains and analyse these for possible chromosomal abnormalities which cause conditions like Down's syndrome. The risk of Down's syndrome increases with the age of the mother, gradually up to the age of 39 and rapidly over 40 (see p. 101). It is the most serious risk facing an older mother. Amniocentesis is often recommended for all pregnant women over 40 and in some areas 39 or even 35.

Availability The decision as to who is offered amniocentesis depends on balancing the risks against the probability of finding an abnormality. Not a routine test, amniocentesis will probably be recommended for you if:

1 you are over 39 or 40;
2 there is a family history (in either partner) of any clearly identifiable congenital or genetic defect;
3 you already have an abnormal child;
4 you are a known or suspected carrier for serious sex-linked diseases such as Duchenne, muscular dystrophy or haemophilia.

Risks The risks of amniocentesis are assessed by a multicentre Medical Research Council study to be under 1 per cent.[5] The major risk to you is of spontaneous abortion following the procedure and it may be a risk you are not prepared to take if it has been difficult to become pregnant. Some surveys rate the risk slightly higher but they tend to consider any pregnancy that goes wrong after 16 weeks to be a direct result of the amniocentesis, which might not be the case. There are some other risks: fetomaternal haemorrhage, which can lead to haemolytic disease (the classical form of which is the 'Rhesus baby' problem); infection; damage to the baby; or chronic leakage of liquor resulting in deformities. However, these are rare. A survey in the *British Medical Journal* in 1978 put the overall risk at between 0.3 and 0.7 per cent.[6]

How it works The test is carried out when you are 16 weeks pregnant. Before that there are not enough fetal cells in the amniotic fluid to provide an accurate analysis. An ultrasound scan will be made first to locate the exact position of the placenta and the fetus, to determine whether it is a single or multiple pregnancy and to establish and mark the site for the needle.

In the test itself a fine hollow needle is inserted into the lower part of the abdomen and about 20 cc of amniotic fluid (a test-tube full) is withdrawn. The fluid is replaced very quickly by the body. Most women say that amniocentesis is not very painful – it is done in the hospital outpatient department and you can eat beforehand and can walk or drive afterwards. It is recommended, however, that you shouldn't do any heavy lifting straightaway.

The cells are cultured in a specialist laboratory, often in a different hospital, and a chromosomal analysis is done. This is a slow, skilled and expensive procedure. Any chromosomal abnormality will be shown up and a diagnosis can then be made on the developing fetus. The chromosome analysis will also determine the sex of the baby but unless the disorder for which they are searching depends on the sex of the fetus the laboratory reserves the right not to disclose this information. (This is because of the supposedly growing number of people who are seeking this test solely to pick the sex of their baby.) If the information is available it is then up to each couple to decide whether or not they would like to know in advance whether their baby is a boy or a girl.

The analysis of the test takes about three weeks as the cultures must have time to grow. As Kay says below, this is commonly felt to be the worst aspect of amniocentesis. It is quite natural to be apprehensive about the outcome of the test and worth reminding yourself that 95 per cent of fetuses are completely healthy.

On the day, I drove myself to the hospital. For the actual amniocentesis I was asked to lie on my back and relax – impossible with so much at stake. I am not a good patient at the best of times, but find it helps if I know what is going on. So I asked lots of questions and was annoyed to receive some very condescending replies, as if it was really not my business what was going on at the lower end of my abdomen.

One thing that worried me slightly was the risk of a miscarriage after an amniocentesis, especially if the needle penetrated the placenta. The doctor reassured me on this point by using a small scanning machine to locate the placenta. When he was sure the placenta was not going to be in the way, he decided where to insert the needle and gave me a local anaesthetic. The insertion of the needle wasn't painful, but was decidedly unpleasant; I could feel the pressure on the inner bag containing the amniotic fluid, and then the puncture.

It was over quite quickly and I drove back wondering why I was supposed to need taking home. Later in the day, as the anaesthetic wore off, it did feel painful but this only lasted two or three days. The three weeks following the test were a great strain, as I felt I had to know the results before I dared to tell my friends that I was pregnant; and it was beginning to show! The two main tests were for spina bifida and mongolism and I had to ring after one week and three weeks for the results. The spina bifida test was OK and my hand shook as I dialled again two weeks later for the mongolism test results. All clear. At last we felt we could actually plan on having this baby.

Accuracy It is worth considering quite carefully what you would do if an abnormality is found. Within the realm of known defects that can be diagnosed from this test, e.g. Down's syndrome or spina bifida, the diagnostic accuracy of amniocentesis is very high. Few mistakes are made and there are very few false-positive diagnoses. If it is shown that there are chromosomal abnormalities in the fetus, a termination will be offered.

If you decide that a termination is what you want, it will probably be a very distressing time for you and you will need a great deal of support. The feelings of guilt and of grieving that many women feel after any termination are sometimes unexpected when they come. If you feel that you would not be prepared to undergo a termination of pregnancy under any circumstances, it is important to think very carefully about your feelings before embarking on this type of investigation. The majority of parents would, under these conditions, prefer not to know of any abnormality but others feel that prior warning of the problems they are to face will help them to prepare for the difficult task of caring for a handicapped child. Most obstetricians and genetic counsellors will respect these wishes and offer the test.

A possible alternative A new technique for obtaining fetal cells for chromosome analysis is being developed. This involves passing a fine needle through the mother's abdominal wall or up through the cervix under ultrasound guidance and sampling the edge of the forming placenta. *Chorionic villus sampling* has two important advantages over amniocentesis. First, it can be performed in the first three months of pregnancy and second, the culture time for the cells is much shorter. Together these allow the detection of a chromosomal abnormality early enough for simpler and safer termination of an affected pregnancy. The technique is still in its infancy, however, and there is inadequate information about the overall risks of the procedure.

Rhesus blood groups

About 15 per cent of people in Britain have a Rhesus-negative blood group. If Rhesus-positive blood enters their bloodstream, antibodies develop and retain the capacity to destroy Rhesus-positive blood cells whenever they enter the bloodstream in the future. These antibodies can also cross over the placenta into the fetus during a pregnancy and cause a syndrome of anemia, heart failure and, in severe cases, intrauterine death – the Rhesus baby syndrome.

If you have a Rhesus-negative blood group, testing for antibodies will be repeated several times during the pregnancy to ensure that there is no risk of this problem developing. The most common cause of this mixing of incompatible bloods is the almost inevitable mixing of some blood from the placenta with the mother's blood at the time of delivery. It is therefore unusual to find antibodies present during a first pregnancy. This may occur, however, if an incompatible blood transfusion has been given in the past or an early spontaneous abortion has gone unnoticed.

Older mothers carry a slightly higher risk of developing antibodies during a pregnancy as this unusual event may follow abnormal bleeding in pregnancy – a threatened abortion or an antepartum haemorrhage – both more common in women over 30. Or it may be a complication of amniocentesis or external cephalic version (turning of the fetus by gentle pressure on the maternal abdomen).

Reaction occurs only when the baby is Rhesus-positive and the mother Rhesus-negative. The initial formation of antibodies can be prevented if a protective injection of 'Anti-D' immunoglobulin is given to the mother within three days of the delivery of her baby. The baby's blood group is established by taking a sample of blood, usually from the placenta. If the baby is Rhesus-positive, the injection is then offered in order to prevent problems in the next pregnancy. Unfortunately, if antibodies have already formed there is at present no way of removing them.

Biochemical tests of placental function

If there is a possibility that your baby is growing more slowly than expected in the uterus, a number of biochemical tests to gauge the efficiency of the placenta may be recommended. The one most commonly employed is to measure a group of hormones normally called 'oestriols', made by the combined effort of the mother, placenta and the fetus. A proportion of this production passes back to the mother and is present in her blood and urine. Depending on the method used in different centres, the test may involve a blood test, taken at a specific time of day, or a collection of urine over a period of up to 24 hours. The latter can be done at home. Other hormones, particularly human placental lactogen (HPL) may be tested for. In each case there is a wide variation of the normal pattern of hormone levels so the results act only as a guide to the welfare of your baby and are used in conjunction with other tests such as ultrasound, fetal movement counting and cardiotocography.

Fetal movement counting

There is an increasing interest in what a baby is able to 'tell' its mother and hence, by those caring for a pregnancy, in the pattern of normal daily activity before birth. Most babies settle into patterns of movement in the last three months of a pregnancy and sudden cessation of movement, or dramatic quieting of the baby may be a warning that all is not well. In order to use this information more objectively, you may be asked to keep a record of the way your baby moves – either how many movements occur in a certain length of time or the length of time taken to achieve a given number of movements. The results can be entered on a chart – often called a 'kick chart' – and taken to antenatal checks. This would be towards the end of your pregnancy.

Every baby behaves differently and the interest in the results is not in comparing one chart with another, but watching your baby's pattern as it emerges. The process is simple, cheap and harmless although it depends on you being both honest and accurate in keeping the record if it is to be helpful. Most women enjoy taking an active part in their antenatal monitoring, but some find it rather stressful and prefer not to do it.

Cardiotocography

In many hospital departments the wellbeing of the baby is also assessed by recording the baby's heart rate over a period of 20–30 minutes. This is achieved by a monitoring machine that uses ultrasound to detect the heartbeat and produces a printed record. When a healthy fetus moves about in the uterus, or is squeezed by the normal painless contractions of late pregnancy, she responds by an increase in heart rate. This is akin to the effect of exercise on the pulse rate of an adult. If the baby is receiving a diminished oxygen supply from the placenta, she may be unable to respond normally to this stimulus and the pattern may become flat, or occasionally the heart rate fall.

The object of this test is to identify a baby who is becoming distressed. If there is a sudden weight loss or there seems to be a temporary slowing down in the baby's activity, it can be helpful to be able to make a rapid check on the baby's wellbeing.

Termination of Pregnancy

If any of your antenatal tests show that the baby you are carrying is likely to be deformed or handicapped, you can ask for a termination of pregnancy. Therapeutic abortion or termination of pregnancy is legal in Britain until up to 28 weeks of pregnancy on a number of specific grounds. Contracting rubella in the first three months of pregnancy, an AFP test that led to the demonstration of spina bifida or other neural tube defect, an amniocentesis which showed a chromosomal abnormality like Down's syndrome, would all constitute legal grounds.

Methods

The choice of operation usually depends on how far advanced the pregnancy is. After the first 3–4 months of pregnancy the contents of the uterus can usually be removed by dilating the cervix and sucking out the fetus through a narrow tube. The operation is usually carried out under general anaesthetic although in the very early weeks this may not be necessary. If abortion is used as a back-up contraception method, it is important to try and have the termination performed as early as possible in the pregnancy.

After the first three months of pregnancy, termination is less simple and a good deal more unpleasant. The safest method currently available involves the injection of drugs which induce the uterus to contract and expel the pregnancy during a process rather like labour.

Effects on a future pregnancy

The vast majority of women having an abortion suffer no adverse effects at the time or in their subsequent pregnancies and there is no evidence that the small risk of problems accelerates with repeated terminations although the risks are present each time. However, if you have had an abortion in the past, do tell your doctor about it so that any possible problems can be anticipated. As has been said already, there may be psychological feelings of guilt and bereavement after a termination that are hard to cope with.

Problems during Pregnancy

As has been said, a healthy woman, whatever her age, is likely to have a straightforward pregnancy. However, the majority of problems that may arise become more common and more troublesome as the mother gets older. More problems are encountered in first pregnancies than with second or third babies, after which the difficulties may increase again. In a first pregnancy every woman is an unknown quantity and a greater fuss may be made of minor abnormalities for this reason.

Although only a minority of older women will encounter problems, it may be helpful and reassuring to know of these possibilities. In some instances there may be existing medical problems that will affect the pregnancy. For others, the problems arising may be a part of the pregnancy itself. The majority of problems arise towards the end of an otherwise smooth pregnancy but a different group of abnormalities can occur in the early months.

The early months

Fibroids Fibroids are harmless muscular lumps in the walls of the uterus. They are quite common – about 20 per cent of women will have fibroids by the time they reach the menopause. The older you are the more likely you are to have fibroids.

Although normally slow-growing, they may increase rapidly during a pregnancy, often the first sign that you have them. They don't harm the baby but occasionally cause problems by becoming tender or painful. If at the bottom of the uterus they may obstruct labour, making a Caesarean section necessary. The majority of women with fibroids are able to have a normal delivery although blood loss at birth is often greater than average as the uterus does not shrink so efficiently afterwards. After the birth, fibroids nearly always shrink down considerably and seldom cause any problems in the future.

Ectopic pregnancy In this uncommon condition, the fertilized ovum is implanted outside the wall of the uterus, usually in one of the Fallopian tubes. The pregnancy cannot develop normally and either dies or ruptures. The latter can be dangerous and requires an operation to rectify it. The condition is not directly related to maternal age but is more common when there is existing pelvic inflammatory disease. An ectopic pregnancy can also occur if an IUCD is in place as this does not prevent implantation in the tube.

Spontaneous abortion Spontaneous abortion, or miscarriage, is a good deal more common than is often realized. At least 10 per cent and possibly as many as 25 per cent of all pregnancies end in miscarriage and the rates rise with maternal age. Most miscarriages occur in the first three months of pregnancy.

It is estimated that between 20 and 40 per cent of spontaneous abortions are caused by a chromosomal abnormality in the fetus, regardless of age of mother or father. Since older women have a greater risk of producing a fetus with chromosomal abnormalities (see p. 99) this is one of the reasons for the increased rates of miscarriage. Another may possibly be more erratic hormone control. Older women with a history of subfertility may have some underlying problem that makes them more vulnerable to miscarriage. Whatever the reason, a woman over 35 is almost twice as likely to miscarry as a woman in her early twenties.

Spacing pregnancies is also a factor. If conception occurs within three months of a spontaneous abortion, there is an increased risk of recurrence. An older woman, feeling that time is running out, may not feel able to wait long enough and therefore could miscarry again. It has been shown that both alcohol and smoking have an effect on miscarriage. The incidence is twice as high in smokers than in non-smokers. The condition known as the 'blighted ovum' is also more common in older women. The placental tissue develops normally but there is no fetus. This usually ends in spontaneous abortion before 16 weeks.

Even though spontaneous abortions are comparatively common, they are still extremely distressing for the women who have them. It often means hospitalization and in some hospitals women who are miscarrying are placed in the same ward as pregnant women or women who have already given birth, which can add to the pain and sadness. It may be necessary to have a D & C (dilitation and curettage – a 'scrape') after a miscarriage to make sure that the uterus is quite empty. For an older woman there may be the added anxiety that she will not be able to have a child at all after she has miscarried. Monica had her first child at 34, became pregnant again when Jane was nine months old and then miscarried.

> I felt an overpowering sense of loss – felt bereft. I wrote to the gynaecologist at the hospital thanking him for his concern and sympathy. That freed my anger against the hospital but I had a fantasy of smashing up the theatre, skulking around dustbins looking for my fetus. Inwardly I was angrily demanding it back again. I was aware of feeling powerful anger at someone and that it had not been justified. That was natural but irrational. I finally accepted that it had to be and anger gave way to depression.

Six months later she was pregnant again, this time successfully, but the experience stays with her.

Other health problems

Anemia If you have a tendency towards anemia, this could get worse during pregnancy. The fetus obtains the considerable supplies of iron and folic acid that she needs from the mother, so you might need to supplement your intake of iron and folic acid during pregnancy. However, if you have a good mixed diet and were not anemic before pregnancy, the supplements are not necessary.

High blood pressure Raised blood pressure (hypertension) becomes more common as people get older. There may be no signs to indicate that this is happening until the level becomes dangerously high, so this is a good reason on its own for regular checks. In most cases there is no apparent cause for the increase in blood pressure – this is known as *essential hypertension*. If you already have even mildly elevated blood pressure, this may give rise to concern during your pregnancy because there is evidence to show that the growth of the fetus may be retarded if the mother's blood pressure is high. If the level is high enough to be a danger to mother or fetus, the blood pressure can be lowered artificially with drugs.

Pre-eclampsia Unlike essential hypertension, in this condition the blood pressure is normal at the start of pregnancy and rises to an abnormal level in the last three months. In addition oedema may occur (swelling of the ankles, fingers or face) and an accumulation of protein in the urine. If very severe it may progress to *eclampsia*, in which convulsions occur. This condition, although now very rare, is dangerous to both mother and baby.

Pre-eclampsia is the most common variety of what used to be called 'toxaemia'. It is more common in first pregnancies and the incidence increases in women over 30. The cause of this condition is known but it is believed that the signs noted in the mother, who may herself feel well, are a consequence of a deterioration in the condition of the placenta or the fetus and may indicate a lack of nutrition and oxygen supply to the fetus. This, in turn, retards the growth of the baby *in utero*.

Diabetes Diabetes is one of the most prevalent metabolic diseases and has been increasing, perhaps because of the increase of sugar in our diet. There are two distinct groups of diabetics: those who need insulin injections and who usually develop the disease when they are young; and the more common non-insulin dependent diabetics who develop problems in middle or old age. If you are already diabetic you will need to talk to your doctor about controllng your blood–sugar level throughout the pregnancy. Control of both forms of diabetes is important as very high levels of blood–sugar can damage the fetus. Also, a baby born to a mother with poorly controlled diabetes may have difficulty controlling her own blood–sugar level for the first two days of life and will need intensive care.

There is another form of diabetes in pregnancy which is of particular interest to older women as the incidence rises with age. This 'gestational diabetes' is present only during pregnancy and disappears after the birth. It may be revealed by finding glucose in the urine, an unusually large baby or the presence of an excessive amount of amniotic fluid. Treatment is usually by controlling carbohydrates in the diet alone, although very rarely insulin may be necessary.

Thyroid problems Either an overactive thyroid (hyperthyroidism) or an underactive thyroid (hypothyroidism) are both associated with subfertility, so a woman with thyroid problems may take some time to become pregnant and therefore be older when she succeeds. Both conditions require careful supervision during pregnancy.

Multiple pregnancy Once a woman is over 35 there is a higher than average chance that she will have twins, although the likelihood is greater the more children she has. The majority of twins are fraternal ones, formed by the fertilization of two separate ova each by a separate sperm. This results in two individuals with different genetic composition, no more alike than siblings. Identical twins are much less common, occurring in 1 in 250 pregnancies. The incidence does not increase significantly with maternal age but there is a slight hereditary trend so the chances are increased if another member of the family has identical twins.

The presence of twins or occasionally even higher numbers of babies can be detected early in pregnancy by ultrasound scanning. Suspicion may arise on clinical examination if the uterus is unusually large for the stage of the pregnancy. Multiple pregnancies receive careful antenatal attention because although there are not usually any special problems, any complications of pregnancy may be more dramatic.

Antepartum haemorrhage Any bleeding occurring in pregnancy is abnormal and should not be ignored. In the majority of cases there is no sinister reason for slight blood loss but the more important abnormalities must be ruled out.

Placenta praevia The placenta normally implants and forms in the fundus of the uterus, the muscular upper half. If the site of the placenta is lower than usual it may encroach on the cervix, or cover it and obstruct the progress of labour. In this abnormal position bleeding always occurs, either in pregnancy or in labour and a Caesarean section may be necessary. There is an increase in the incidence of *placenta praevia* with maternal age, especially over 35, but the link is stronger if the woman has already had several children and particularly if she is malnourished.

Accidental haemorrhage Occasionally there may be bleeding from a normally sited placenta, a condition known as accidental haemorrhage or placental abruption. Since this bleeding causes the separation of the placenta from the wall of the uterus, it cuts off part of the oxygen supply to the fetus and can jeopardize the life of the baby and perhaps the mother. If a small bleed of this type occurs but the pregnancy is allowed to continue, the growth of the fetus will be carefully monitored to ensure that oxygen and nutritional supplies are adequate. The risk of accidental haemorrhage is higher in older women but those with poor social circumstances, those who smoke and those with several previous pregnancies are at greater risk.

Since both *placenta praevia* and accidental haemorrhage are serious conditions, you would be asked to report immediately if any vaginal bleeding occurs in the last four months of pregnancy.

Planning and Preparation during Pregnancy

When you are pregnant it can be difficult to see beyond the time of the birth and to accept in a real sense that after it's all over, there is actually going to be a baby at the end of it.

In spite of what might feel like a resistance to thinking too far ahead, just 'in case', there are various things you can usefully do to make life easier for you when the baby does arrive.

The birth

In addition to reading books like this about pregnancy and childbirth, you will probably also go to some classes. *Antenatal classes* are often available in general practices, health centres and clinics and if you are giving birth in hospital, there will be antenatal classes there. Sometimes the level of those classes isn't quite what you want or expect. Aleid:

I went to the hospital class once and then stopped. I didn't think there was anything I could learn there. Although we did some exercises that I thought could be useful, I could also have picked them up from a book. It was all very much about rigid role divisions between husband and wife – you could get your husband to clean the windows for you and do the hoovering. It was a bit low level and patronizing. We were all 'girls'. The teacher would sit there separately as the teacher and there were we – the girls. It was really funny actually. It was clear that she taught the same things all the time, had probably done that for 20 years and hadn't changed a word of it.

Even if this is so, classes do give you a good opportunity to meet other women who may be having a baby at the same time as you. It is good to be able to go and visit another new mother while you are in hospital, rather than waiting for all the visitors to come to you. In the early weeks after the baby is born you will probably be obsessed with the details of feeding and sleeping, weight gain and nappies and it is reassuring to be able to share it with someone else who also feels like that.

You might find the classes organized by the *National Childbirth Trust* (NCT) a more helpful way of finding out what it might be like and learning exercises and techniques for coping with your own labour. Again, it is a good way of meeting other mothers, some of whom may be having second or third babies. Aleid much preferred those: 'NCT was different. It was nice because it was just in somebody's house and you were just sitting around being women together. I found it very good. I enjoyed being there with other women who were pregnant, to share it and talk about it.' The NCT classes also involve fathers in varying degrees and this is important too. The emphasis tends to be on women preparing for birth in most respects but men need to prepare too – not just to help their partners but to talk, with other men, about how they feel about becoming a father. Too often all the information fathers get is filtered through a woman, usually their own partners, and I think they need more than this.

Depending on where you live, other classes may be on offer too. Active Birth Centres, for example, in London, Birmingham, Bangor and Bath offer classes of their own. Aleid also felt that continuing with *yoga for exercise* had helped her:

I was about three months pregnant when I started doing yoga again. I have a very good teacher and had so much confidence in her that I just followed when she said – you don't do this or do that up to there. So I did shoulder stands and head stands with my big belly. I did a lot of those stretching exercises. During the delivery it was the natural thing to squat and move my bottom around and it just came naturally. The midwife said I had a very flexible spine and I think that must have been the yoga.

The emphasis put on flexibility of movement and particularly on relaxation makes yoga an excellent form of exercise to do during pregnancy as long as you have a teacher you trust.

Things to make life easier

You will almost certainly be aware, particularly towards the end of your pregnancy, that you won't have much time to yourself that is free from responsibility for a long time. There may be all sorts of things it would be helpful to do or find out before the baby comes.

- If you can afford to *stock up on basic household items*, this is a good time to do it. Apart from bulky or heavy things like loo paper, washing powder, etc., it is worth having a hoard of tasty, nourishing things you like to eat and that will make quick, convenient snacks that are also good for you after the baby is born – sardines, peanut butter, dried fruit, nuts, granola bars, etc.
- If you have a freezer (or can borrow some space in someone else's) you could *stock up on prepared meals* that will save time and energy. If they are also things that can be eaten with one hand while you hold the baby in the other arm, so much the better!
- Babies are big business. It is very easy to be seduced by the very attractive equipment and clothes on the market. But *don't buy too much*. You will be amazed at how much you are given or lent and it is a waste to spend a lot of money on equipment you might not need for very long. Most babies are out of their first-size clothing long before the advertised three months is up.
- Find out about *second-hand* baby equipment shops in your area and start looking at adverts in local newspapers and shop windows. Well-baby clinics have noticeboards where people advertise items for sale too. If you can, borrow things you will need for a short time only – like a crib or a baby bouncer. Some things, second-hand cots in particular, are in great demand so it is worth starting to look early. The cost of new cots is horrifying: £75–100.
- If you can afford to get *one new piece of equipment* it is probably worth buying your own pushchair or buggy. They get a great deal of use from six months onwards and a good one will make

your life a lot easier. But don't buy it now – wait until you have been out and about with your baby for a few months and can weigh up the pros and cons of the different types available.

● *Talk to people* you know who have small children and find out what they found useful, necessary, essential. Ask about clothes too.

● People have surprisingly strong views about *nappies* and no doubt you will develop them too. Not just about what goes into them but which kind is best. You will find people who swear by disposable nappies and others who found that disposables gave their babies a rash and preferred terry-towelling ones. All nappies are expensive, so if you are at all unsure about what sort to use, get a range of different kinds to try in the first couple of weeks before deciding. You can borrow a few terry nappies. If you spend over £25 on new terry nappies you might feel bound to use them even if you find disposables suit you better.

● You will certainly use nappy liners, zinc and castor oil cream and cotton wool, so get plenty in advance.

● *Get to know some babies* in your neighbourhood. If you know someone whose baby was born a few months before yours, she could be very helpful. She won't have forgotten all the useful bits of information you want to know.

Time for yourself

It is well worth planning ahead to see that you are going to get a break from the baby on a regular basis so you can do something for yourself. Giving birth and looking after a small baby is an exhausting business, not just physically but emotionally too. The strong feelings you have for your baby and the swings of mood that are common after the birth drain your mental energy. You need to put back some of that energy, and one of the ways of doing that is to find something you really like doing for yourself that has nothing to do with the baby. That is where you operate as you, not a mother. It might mean going for a walk, painting, reading, cycling, going to yoga or some other class, joining a group, going out for a drink with your partner or for a meal with a friend. Think now how you could organize something regularly quite soon after the birth:

1 Are there friends who would occasionally look after the

baby for a short while between feeds, either at your house or theirs?

2 Can your partner create a regular slot when he is prepared to take charge?

3 Can you take the baby with you?

When should you stop working?

This is entirely up to you. Maternity regulations provide for you to give up work 11 weeks before the baby is due but there is no need to do this if you don't want to. If you are fit and well and happy to continue with your job, that is your choice. If, on the other hand, you are getting very tired, aren't sleeping well because you aren't comfortable and constantly have to wake up to go to the loo, it might be worth stopping work. Make sure that your blood pressure is checked regularly and get advice if your hands or ankles start swelling up. It is a good thing to be as well and as rested as possible before you go into labour. If you are planning to go back to work fairly soon after the birth, you can usually take the 11 weeks you are entitled to before the birth after the baby is born instead. But you might lose some of your maternity allowance (see p. 65).

While you are deciding when to stop work, it is worth thinking about *how you will spend those weeks*. You might have lots of things you want to do and be happy doing them – what my partner called 'nest-building' when I did that. On the other hand it can be a lonely time if you are already well-organized and most of your friends are at work. You could find that several weeks off work can be unsettling, that time hangs heavily and you have too much time to brood and worry. Or it can be simply boring. Angela found it so:

> Things became a little flat at home when I left work. I swelled enormously until I looked like one of those large beach balls. I tried to kill time by taking long country walks and reading various babycare paperbacks, but all I wanted was for my baby to arrive. I had my suitcase packed for the hospital by week 35. A sense of anti-climax was setting in by week 40.

If your baby doesn't arrive on time, as is very common, you might find it even harder to wait that bit longer than you expected. Another woman felt she had made a mistake in the last few weeks of her pregnancy, by doing everything in the house and getting a meal ready each evening – her partner really expected her to go on doing it afterwards too. After all, it was 'only' a baby who had joined them.

It may be possible to *leave the final decision* about when to stop work to see how you feel. If you can do this, it might be better not to commit yourself in advance.

Maternity Benefits

Maternity grant

This is a sum of £25 paid to help with the immediate costs of having a baby. It is the lowest maternity grant in Europe. Every mother is entitled to it, whether single or married and irrespective of National Insurance contributions. *When to claim*: Nine weeks before the baby is due up until three months after the birth. Get form BM4 from your maternity or child-welfare clinic or the Social Security office. You also need Mat.B1, the certificate of expected confinement signed by your midwife, health visitor or doctor.

Maternity allowance

This is a weekly payment of a sum the same as Unemployment Benefit, payable for 18 weeks as long as you are not doing paid work. You are entitled to the allowance whether you are single or married as long as you have paid National Insurance contributions for two years. You may also be entitled to it if you have been paying contributions for slightly less time but maternity allowance can only be claimed on your own insurance. It is paid for *11 weeks before* the birth and *7 weeks afterwards* as long as you are not working. If you go on working after the eleventh week before your due date, you will probably not be paid the full allowance. If your baby is late, claim for each additional week after your estimated date of delivery. *When to claim*: Not before 14 weeks and not later than 11 weeks before the baby is due. Get the claim form BM4 from your clinic or the Social Security office. You will also need Mat.B1, the certificate of expected confinement.

Maternity pay

If you qualify for this you will get paid for at least six weeks after you leave work. The money will be payable by your employer and you will get 90 per cent of your basic pay, less the state maternity allowance. You are entitled to maternity pay if you satisfy the following conditions:

1 you must have been employed continuously by the same employer for at least two years at the beginning of the eleventh week before the baby is due;
2 you must normally work at least 16 hours a week;
3 you must still be employed at the beginning of the eleventh week before the baby is due;
4 you must notify your employer 21 days before you stop work or as soon as is practicable that you will be stopping work because of pregnancy or confinement;
5 if the employer asks, you must provide a certificate signed by your doctor or midwife giving the estimated date of the baby's birth.

Six weeks' maternity pay is the statutory minimum. It is possible that your contract gives a longer period of paid leave after a shorter qualification time, so it is worth checking the contract wording. For your rights at work, see p. 207.

● Depending on your circumstances, you may be able to claim *Unemployment Benefit*. To be eligible for Unemployment Benefit you must be 'available for work'. This means that you might have to provide proof that you have made arrangements for childcare before you sign on. A new test for availability is being introduced after the Rayner Report (1980) singled out 'married women with young children' as seeing Unemployment Benefit as a source of easy money.

You can claim Unemployment Benefit if you are out of work as long as you have paid full National Insurance contributions for the relevant period, i.e. in the last complete tax year before the calendar year in which you claim (e.g. to claim from January 1985 onwards, you must have contributions in the tax year from April 1983 to April 1984). The standard rate of benefit is paid until you have been claiming it for a full year, then it stops. If you get work for at least 13 weeks and work for at least 16 hours a week, and if you then become unemployed again, you should be able to claim benefit for another year. *How to claim*: Go to your local Employment Office or Job Centre after the baby is born and register for work. Your maternity allowance will stop after seven weeks and you may register any time after that. Take with you the P45 (the income tax form your employer should have given you when you left work) and your National Insurance number. Then go to the Unemployment Benefit Office to 'sign on' and fill in a form to claim benefit. You will be told to come back to the office each fortnight to sign on.

● *Child benefit* is a sum paid weekly or monthly for each child, to which everybody is entitled. You get an allowance book after the baby is born and collect the money from the Post Office or have it paid directly into your bank account. If you are a single parent you are entitled to an additional sum per child per week.

Other benefits

Free prescriptions You can get free prescriptions if you are pregnant and until the baby is one year old. Ask your doctor, midwife or health visitor for a claim form and send it to the Family Practitioner Committee.

Free dental treatment If you are pregnant or have had a baby in the past year you can get free dental treatment. Tell the dentist you are pregnant and you will be given a form to sign.

Free milk and vitamins If you get Supplementary Benefit or Family Income Supplement you are entitled to free milk and vitamins. You get tokens for seven pints of milk a week (which you give to your milkman), two bottles of vitamin drops every three months and vitamin drops for your baby. If you have a low income fill in the form on the leaflet 'Free Milk and Vitamins' from a Post Office and send it to the Social Security Office.

Fares to hospital If you have a low income or get Supplementary Benefit or Family Income Supplement you can get help with fares to the hospital when you go for antenatal or postnatal visits.

Supplementary Benefit If you cannot get a maternity allowance and you have no one to support you or your maternity allowance isn't enough to live on, you can claim Supplementary Benefit. You cannot claim if you are married and living with your husband or if you are living with a man 'as husband and wife'. If you are, it is the man who must make the claim. He will receive the rate for a married man which is less than the rate for two single people. A great deal of hardship results from this rule, formerly known as the 'cohabitation rule' when it is applied to a single woman who lives with a man but wishes to be financially independent. If you are entitled to Supplementary Benefit, you can claim a single payment to cover the cost of necessary non-medical equipment, e.g. a second-hand cot, pram, maternity clothes, etc. This can be quite a large amount of money. *How to claim*: Fill in form SB1 from a Post Office or the Social Security Office.

Insurance You might want to consider taking out insurance on your life. Quite a lot of men have life insurance or a 'death insurance' linked to their jobs but it is more unusual for women to have life-insurance policies. If you are planning to take the major responsibility for looking after your baby yourself as many women do, it is an interesting exercise to cost what it would mean to employ somebody else to do those jobs, if anything happened to you. For an annual premium of about £15 to £20 you could cover yourself.

4

The Birth

As a woman over 30 you can expect to be treated with care during your labour, especially with your first baby. Because there is a gradual generalized increase in the problems a woman may meet as she gets older, doctors and midwives tend to be on the lookout for the first signs of trouble, however minor. But you may well have a perfectly normal labour and delivery. Your state of general health and fitness, the way you feel about your pregnancy and the way you prepare for the birth can all help counter any effect of age alone.

Intervention

The question of intervention in childbirth has become an area of public concern and controversy. The trend to move childbirth out of the home and into the specialized, technological atmosphere of a hospital has made many women speak out about their experiences and criticisms. The overall picture that has emerged is not always a happy one. As we have already seen, pregnancy and labour are treated as an illness, the mother as a patient. It is as if no one ever had babies safely before.

One of the reasons for the increase of intervention in the process of birth is connected with the way the medical profession evaluates obstetric practice. Perinatal mortality rates are frequently used as the main barometer of efficiency in hospitals and while these are clearly very important (and the rate in Britain is higher than it should be when compared with many other industrialized countries) that is not the only consideration. Nor can we be entirely sure that hospital births are so much safer than well-organized home confinements. Technological innovations have developed so quickly in obstetrics that there have not yet been sufficient studies to prove their effectiveness when used in a routine way and to allay the doubts about some of the side-effects. Also, once hospitals have bought expensive machines and trained people to use them, a rationale can develop for routine use of technology to justify the costs involved.

All the same, public pressure *can* affect what happens and change things. In the last decade organizations like the NCT (National Childbirth Trust) and AIMS (the Association for the Improvement of Maternity Services) have campaigned for women to have more knowledge about and control over the way their babies are born. These attitudes are sometimes seen as dangerous and threatening by a medical profession used to an autonomous and hierarchically organized system. Nevertheless, the exposure in the press in 1974 of very high rates of induction in British hospitals has led to a real decrease in the incidence of inducing labour in many areas. And although there are more babies delivered by Caesarean section in Britain than in Holland and some other European countries, figures are not nearly as high as for the USA and Canada.

Older first-time mothers

There may be a greater readiness to intervene in the labour of a woman over 30 giving birth for the first time – perhaps earlier than is always necessary. If this happens to you it will be because there seems to be a greater risk for you and your baby. What you need in order to feel confident that you are getting the right treatment and advice is information about what is happening to you and an explanation for any course of action suggested to you. It is possible to get detailed general information by reading and talking to people. There is a list of books that deal with the detail of childbirth on p. 215, but you might also ask women you know which books they found helpful. Antenatal classes will give you a good idea of what should happen at a normal birth.

Getting your wishes known

You will probably have some ideas, perhaps strong ones, about what sort of labour you would like and it is worth discussing them with the doctors and midwives you see. If you do have clear ideas and attend a hospital clinic where you don't see the same medical staff each visit, make sure that your wishes are written down in your notes in a prominent way. Or you could write a letter. Julia had a bad experience with her first labour at the age of 35. Shortly before she had her second baby at 39 she wrote a long letter to the matron of the hospital setting out what had gone wrong before. She was impressed by the difference it made. All the midwives attending her had read the letter and 'very nice to me they were too. I don't think I'd have had the nerve,' she said, 'to write a long detailed letter of complaint just before returning to the same place in my twenties.' Being older can give you more confidence in dealing with the authorities and you don't have to wait for things to go wrong before stating what you would like.

Getting information

It is important for you to have the information about your pregnancy and labour necessary to help you exercise your choices completely and confidently. That information, pertaining to *your own* situation and not to some routine procedure for all older women, is the base from which you can understand. If you want to know something, ask. Educating yourself into asking the right sort of questions or knowing what to ask is probably quite important too. One consultant obstetrician told me, 'I always make a point of asking women whether they have any queries and it's surprising how infrequently they ask questions. Whilst I don't view myself as being intimidating, I can understand that women may be reluctant to come out with questions.'

Things you can do

- If you are anxious or puzzled about anything, write it down so you don't forget to ask about it when you have the chance.
- If you have a particular problem (say, heartburn or swollen fingers) think carefully about when it started, anything that causes changes, any information that might help – in other words, monitor yourself.
- If someone gives you an explanation you don't understand (perhaps using medical terminology you don't know) ask to

have it explained further, don't pretend you really understand.
● If you think you are being fobbed off with patronizing or
jokey remarks like 'that baby would be better in the cot', stay
calm and pleasant but ask for reasons.
● If you are unlucky enough to be dealing with a doctor or
midwife who seems to be unhelpful or uncommunicative, ask
to see someone else.

A caution

While it is a good thing to think carefully about where you should
have the baby, the sort of labour you would like and what kind of
help you would like in terms of pain relief, it is worth
remembering that giving birth is a pretty unpredictable business
so it is as well to have a flexible approach.

Birth at home

This chapter assumes that most women over 30 having their first
babies will have them in hospital. Since only one baby in a 100 is
born at home, older women meet great resistance to the idea of
home delivery because of the somewhat higher risk of problems
developing. However, some women do manage to organize a
home confinement, so if that is something you feel strongly
about, follow it up (see p. 42). Annie found that having her
baby at home worked wonderfully well. It was quite a long
labour, about 18 hours, but she felt relaxed and able to do the
things that would help her through it:

> It was lovely. There was a big state of excitement in the house.
> It was a lovely day, really sunny, so I got dressed and we were
> all sitting out in the garden in deck chairs. It was a big party
> and all the neighbours were calling out, 'How are you?' and
> 'What's going on?' I was walking round as much as I could
> through my contractions and Don could massage my back. If
> he wasn't around someone else would do it. . . . Later, if I was
> lying down for an examination the pain was quite unbearable.
> I felt then that if I'd been in hospital and lying down, I
> couldn't have coped with the pain but I could walking round.
> I knew that the hospital was very close if things went wrong. I
> suppose the most important thing for me was the atmosphere
> being right. When she was born, everything was so nice, Don
> and I were very close. It was a very magical feeling.

Birth in hospital

It is easy to forget, in the midst of all the complaints and criticisms, that many women have perfectly normal births in hospital too and feel good about them. Alison had her first baby when she was 33. Her labour was rather shorter than average but in every way it was a completely normal birth.

I have never regarded childbirth as the ultimate experience for a woman but rather as something a woman must go through in order to have a child. As I live in Italy, I decided to have my first child in England. Both Giorgio and I wanted the father present at the birth and this was easier in England. I left Italy at 36 weeks and when a couple of weeks later the doctor said I could be early, I panicked and a phone call brought Giorgio to England on the last day of week 38. He arrived at midnight and I was thrilled – so much so that I must have relaxed – for two hours later something started trickling down my leg. I packed my case and at 3 a.m., disbelieving, I went into hospital.

My father, a local GP, took me to the hospital and introduced me to the midwife and reassured me. I was then examined and told that I was 6 cm dilated. I had to shower, be shaved and have an enema which is my most negative memory of the pre-birth stage. But all the time I had to remind myself that I was going to have a baby and that it was happening to me. There was something very unreal about it. It was all happening too quickly.

I was taken into the delivery room and had my waters broken. I had seen the delivery room at antenatal classes and so knew what to expect. I was also lucky. The registrar did me an excellent turn by telling me that he thought the child would be born between 7 and 9 a.m. Having an idea about the time made a tremendous difference psychologically. I knew the pain would not go on for hours and hours. Giorgio's presence made time go quickly because we had three weeks' gossip to catch up on. There was one bad moment when I needed a bedpan and the stink made me sick and a lot of fresh air deodorant was used. The nursing staff were always at hand though not present, but when I vomited between the first and second stage the midwife wiped me down with a damp flannel.

At ten minutes to seven, after many contractions (some almost unbearable) the midwife came in and said, 'Alison, I go

off at 7.30 and I would like to deliver your child.' That gave me
the final fillip. I had been told that the final stage was like
shitting a grapefruit and with that uppermost in my mind I
started to push. It wasn't easy. I used oxygen, but the staff
were fantastic. After the first real push I asked how many like
that were necessary and they said about six so once again I
had a definite idea of what was happening and how long it
would take. It wasn't perfect as I had an episiotomy but after
the fifth or sixth push the doctor said, 'Are you going to sit up
and see your baby being born?' and that spurred me on to the
last push at 7.17 with the midwife still on duty and this 'thing'
there between my legs.

So mine was a very positive experience. It was not
exhilarating. It is extremely exhausting. And I was very lucky.
Giorgio was present, I had an easy, simple birth, greatly
enhanced by the nursing staff and doctors who were able to
give me definite ideas and thus infinite confidence.

Possible Complications

Since the possibility of complications which may develop in
labour is slightly higher with increasing age, it is worth
understanding a few of the difficulties that may arise. None of
these complications are exclusive to women over 30. If an older
woman does have a difficult birth, this may well be related to a
collection of minor factors rather than one specific problem. As
you read on, don't be put off by some of the experiences some
women have. As with many other aspects of this book (and life!)
it is easier and more compelling to talk about difficulties than
about the things that go well, so sometimes there is a rather
unbalanced overall picture. As with chapter 3 on pregnancy, this
chapter does not deal with all aspects of labour and childbirth,
but concentrates on those of special interest to women over 30.

Duration of labour

The labour of an older woman tends to be a little longer than that
of a woman in her twenties, but only by an hour or two. First
labours also tend to be longer than subsequent ones, regardless of
age. It is likely that the tissues required to stretch and the
muscles required to function may become a little less elastic over
the years.

The process of giving birth is not called labour for nothing. It is hard work, harder physical work than most of us are used to. Fatigue is, in itself, one of the biggest problems to cope with during labour especially when, as often happens, it interferes with a night's sleep – another thing older women may cope with less well. During labour you will probably not feel like eating and the stomach fails to absorb food and fluids properly. For this reason you may well be advised to limit yourself to water and glucose during your labour. The loss of body water in the hothouse atmosphere of most delivery suites and the inevitable loss with breathing patterns used may lead to dehydration. In addition, the energy required by the contracting uterus rapidly consumes the body's supply of glucose and a secondary form of metabolism which burns fat comes into operation. The woman may then become ketotic – she feels headachy and vague, she feels less in control of herself and her labour and the uterus itself works less efficiently, slowing down the process of her labour. Under these conditions an intravenous drip containing a solution of glucose (or dextrose) in water may be used to counteract these effects.

Dysfunctional labour

As mentioned above, the uterus of a woman over 30 may work less efficiently because her muscles are unable to contract so well. These differences are often slight and are minimized by good preparation for labour, especially an ability to relax well. However, in a small number of labours the contractions of the uterus are not properly co-ordinated so that they fail to exert an overall push in the right direction. It is often said that this form of labour, known as 'dysfunctional labour', is more painful than a normal one. This is difficult to prove and may be more a reflection of the tiredness and despondency felt by a woman in labour for some time who sees little apparent progress for her efforts. The conditions of ketosis and dehydration mentioned above may also produce this picture in which the cervix fails to dilate, and their treatment is an important step in its correction.

'*Acceleration*' *of labour* is usually used to restore progress when this has slowed down, most commonly due to dysfunctional uterine activity. In this process, a drug called Syntocinon, a synthetic version of one of the body's own hormones, is given in an intravenous drip. Understandably, many women are not keen on this artificial acceleration. It is usually recommended because doctors and midwives are not happy about long, slow labours especially for a woman seen to be a risk, like an older first-time mother.

It may be possible to avoid acceleration of labour by staying at home for longer during the first part of labour and not going to the hospital too soon. Your contractions may start and then stop again but once you have been admitted, the hospital staff may be reluctant to allow you to remain in labour for many hours. In certain cases where the labour is making little progress, acceleration can benefit the baby (for whom a shorter labour is generally safer) and the mother in perhaps enabling her to avoid a Caesarean section and to reach the second stage of labour before she is too exhausted to push her baby out.

Induction

The decision to bring a pregnancy to an end by the process of induction of labour is a very important one and should never be undertaken lightly. Quite understandably, women would rather go into labour at the time that their baby and uterus dictate and are disappointed if this type of intervention is recommended. It is not possible to provide a comprehensive list of the reasons for which induction could be recommended. As a general guide it should only be used if there is good reason to believe that the baby, or occasionally the mother *and* baby, may come to harm if the pregnancy goes on any longer. Rates of induction have been dropping in many areas compared with the early 1970s when they were very high, but there is still a good deal of regional variation. You could ask the consultant obstetrician or the clinic sister what policy the hospital adopts towards inducing labour. All obstetricians tend to err on the safe side and would prefer to induce labour before serious complications occur rather than correct a more difficult problem, but there are some risks and side-effects with induction itself. If this procedure is advised you should be quite sure that the medical reasons are clearly explained.

Cheryl had to go into hospital a few days before her estimated delivery date because of slightly raised blood pressure. She had, against the odds, arranged to have a home birth, so she was very disappointed to be in hospital and was very much against being induced: 'The registrar pestered me daily with remarks that it was a good sized baby and he'd be better in the cot. I stuck it out against induction until the expected date had passed and then I agreed. I wanted to get out of the place.' Cheryl had mild hypertension and her baby weighed 6 lb 6 oz at birth. 'I felt he'd have been better with another week inside me,' she said. He also developed jaundice severely enough to delay her return home, a factor often associated with induction. If there were pressing medical reasons for inducing Cheryl, they were never explained to her and she has been left with the feeling that she was bullied into accepting unnecessary intervention.

A woman over 30 is more likely than average to be advised to have an induction of labour. Nevertheless, it should not be recommended without a specific reason. The most difficult area is when the baby is late. It helps to be as clear as possible about menstrual dates, not always easy if you have been on the pill. There is an individual variation in the length of a normal pregnancy but in women over 30 there is a marked drop in the efficiency of the placenta after week 41. Placental deficiency may result in fetal distress *in utero* and may be connected with sudden loss of weight in the woman. There are tests to prove postmaturity and to see how well the placenta is functioning, so if you are advised an induction simply because your baby is overdue, you should check that there are indications of postmaturity. Fortunately, more older women seem to deliver early (round about week 38) than very late.

Methods Methods used to induce labour vary from unit to unit and should be adapted to suit the needs of each woman. The object is to make the uterus start contracting in a pattern as close as possible to normal labour, leading to the birth of the baby.

- Pessaries of a drug called prostaglandin (a synthetic form of one of the body's hormones produced naturally in labour) introduced into the vagina to help ripen the cervix. 'Ripening' is the term used to describe the softening and shortening of the cervix which often happens before labour contractions start. Prostaglandin intravaginally may also initiate labour
- An intravenous drip containing prostaglandin or Syntocinon (described earlier in the acceleration of labour). If you have to be on a drip during labour this necessarily restricts movement. You will not be able to walk around much and

may have to lie down. If you had other plans, it may be worth
being prepared for this.
● Artificial rupturing of the membranes (ARM) or breaking
the waters, to release the amniotic fluid in front of the baby's
head. This helps dilatation of the cervix by allowing the baby's
head to come into snug contact with it during contractions. It
probably also encourages the release of the woman's own
prostaglandin hormones. Breaking the waters is not comfortable for the mother and can be painful. There is also some
controversy about ARM because some people believe that it
causes more distress to the fetus.

Occasionally *induction is planned* – a diabetic mother or a baby
with Rhesus disease will need special facilities and it is best then
for the birth to take place when they are most available. Just
occasionally an induction may be planned at your convenience –
for example, if your partner might otherwise miss the birth – but
only if you were going to be induced anyway.

Caesarean section

A woman over 30 is somewhat more likely to have a Caesarean
section than a younger woman. If it is known in advance that
your pelvis is too small for a vaginal delivery or if the baby is in a
breech position and cannot be turned, or if the placenta is
obstructing the cervix, an *elective Caesarean* will be performed, i.e.
one that is arranged for a specific date. It ought to be possible in
that case to have an epidural anaesthetic if you would like it so
that you are awake and can see your baby being born.

An *emergency Caesarean* section will be performed if the labour is
not progressing normally and there are indications of danger for
the mother and, especially, the baby. As in so many other
complications of labour, there may not be one specific pointer to
the need for a Caesarean delivery, but several cumulative
reasons. Again, with older women, doctors may be less prepared
to take risks and therefore operate more readily. In an
emergency, it may be necessary to use a general anaesthetic if
there isn't time for an epidural. However, there may be a
functioning epidural in already which can be topped up for the
operation.

The operation performed is almost always a lower segment
Caesarean section (hence LSCS), which means that the baby is

delivered through a side-to-side incision at the bottom of the uterus where the tissue is less vascular and the subsequent healing stronger than in the upper part of the uterus. To get there the usual approach is through a transverse incision at the bottom of the abdomen which looks neater and is more comfortable in the first few days after the operation than the alternative of an up-and-down incision in the skin. The operation takes between 30 and 60 minutes depending on the circumstances, but the baby is born within the first ten minutes; the rest is putting things back together. From the baby's point of view, delivery by LSCS is usually less traumatic than a vaginal delivery but from the mother's it is a major operation which involves inevitable bleeding, the risks of anaesthesia and analgesia and a permanent slight weakness in the wall of the uterus. Also, immediately after the operation the bladder and bowel may function less efficiently; difficulty in mobility carries the risk of deep-vein thrombosis (DVT) and makes looking after the baby more problematic. Women are bullied to get back on their feet and move about because of the DVT risks.

After a Caesarean section it is important to understand clearly the reasons for the operation, not only for the sake of peace of mind but because of what it means for a future pregnancy. Some problems, e.g. a contracted pelvis, will always be a problem. Others, for example a breech presentation, acute fetal distress, are 'non-recurring' and, if the next pregnancy is normal, a vaginal delivery may be possible with safety. If the labour was slow and the baby appeared to get stuck, X-rays of the pelvis may be advised after delivery so that information about the dimensions and shape of the pelvis are available in a future pregnancy.

Monitoring equipment

Since the early 1970s there has been a rapid increase in the use of electronic equipment to monitor the progress of labour and the wellbeing of the fetus. In some hospitals it is now routine to use such equipment for every labour and its use has almost replaced the midwife's stethoscope. The routine use of expensive, specialized equipment is the subject of controversy amongst some obstetricians as well as the general public. Machines are only as good as the person reading them and should not be used without regular assessment of the woman's condition by an experienced midwife. Machines can break down and they are not always accurate. They might fail to pick up signs a midwife might be aware of if she were fully responsible for the progress of the labour. There are rare but alarming cases of hospital staff failing to believe the monitor readings and assuming the machine is faulty, with tragic results.

Kay felt that being monitored was not in her best interests:

> I felt very well at the start although the hospital were concerned about blood pressure. The midwife insisted that I lie on the bed and have attached 1) a monitor for the baby's heart, 2) a belt to measure contractions and 3) a drip in case I needed drugs. In spite of asking if I could remain mobile as I felt so much in command of my labour, the staff used what I now consider moral blackmail to get me to agree. The monitor was for the sake of the baby – if it should become distressed they would know immediately. I began to find the whole process very uncomfortable as I could not move freely so reluctantly agreed to an epidural because my blood pressure was high. Meanwhile, my husband, who had been asked to watch the monitor and is quite experienced in the use of machinery, thought it was not working properly. It did not seem to be measuring contractions correctly, although I was feeling them getting stronger (the epidural only worked on one side) the machine was not reading this. The staff would not listen.

Eventually the machine *was* found to be faulty but not in time to avoid an emergency Caesarean section. Kay is convinced that less dependence on the monitor might have enabled her to give birth more easily.

Many women feel uneasy about the use of monitoring equipment. There is a feeling that its presence dehumanizes labour and indeed there do seem to be occasions when the machine appears to get more attention than the woman.

How it works The monitoring machine records the fetal heart rate either by the use of ultrasound pulses through the mother's abdominal wall or by picking up the electrical impulses through an electrode applied to the baby's head. There is a very slight risk of infection or of damage to the baby with an internal monitor. The *main problem* women used to experience, as Kay described, was that the attachment of the monitoring equipment restricted mobility, especially walking around. It usually meant that the woman had to lie on her back which may have been uncomfortable and not her chosen birth position. This is less common now. It is usually possible to remain upright while being monitored and new design of equipment, especially scalp electrodes, makes women much more mobile than they used to be.

Some women *find it reassuring* to watch their baby's heart rate beating through the labour. It is also possible to turn the sound up and *hear* the heart beat which can be exciting. Contractions register on the monitor as wavy lines so your partner can take a more active part in your labour by watching for the start of a new contraction, telling you when it is coming and so helping you to adjust your breathing. Of course, you will be able to *feel* the contraction (unless you have had an epidural) but it is a concrete way he can help.

Many women and some obstetricians feel that technical equipment is now used more widely than necessary. The midwife using her time-honoured stethoscope can watch over most babies efficiently. Even this technique is safer than it was before the use of fetal heart monitors, as experience of observing the baby continuously has widened knowledge of the danger signs and allows the midwife to use her skills to greater advantage. The supporters of 'monitoring for all' justify their enthusiasm for monitoring as many babies as possible by the fact that about half the babies who become distressed during labour give no warning signs during the antenatal period that all is not well within the uterus. So although the total number of babies at risk is small, timely intervention may save a life or prevent serious damage occurring.

It should be possible for you to have some choice in the matter of monitoring if your labour is running smoothly. Certainly if the machinery is uncomfortable, annoying or upsetting, you should not be afraid to say so. Hospital staff tend to be sensitive about taking risks with older mothers so there will probably be fairly strong pressure to be monitored some of the time.

Episiotomy

The majority of women having their first baby have an episiotomy – an incision made in the perineum (the muscular wall around the back of the vagina) to make it easier to deliver the baby's head. The older you are the more likely it is that you will have an episiotomy because the skin around the vagina does not stretch so easily as you get older.

The reasons given for having an episiotomy are that:

1 it enables the baby to be born more quickly if there are signs of fetal distress;
2 a deliberate cut in a safe place heals better than the alternative, a tear in the vaginal wall where the tissues give way at their weakest point;
3 it helps to prevent weakness and prolapse of the vaginal wall in later life.

However, *doubts have arisen* about some of the arguments, notably in a study of 1,795 women carried out by the National Childbirth Trust: 65 per cent of the women who had vaginal deliveries had an episiotomy. The effects of this most common surgical operation ('the only surgery likely to be performed without her consent on the body of a healthy woman in Western Society'[1]) have received little attention so far. It is often painless at the time but the stitching is often uncomfortable and can cause considerable pain for some time after the birth, making walking, sitting and, therefore, breastfeeding uncomfortable. The NCT study suggests that a tear is less painful than a deliberate cut and heals more quickly. This may be because if there is a tear, the skin and the vagina will tear but probably the muscle will not, so there might be slightly less tissue damage. It may also be easier to put up with something that happens naturally, like a tear, than something that has been done to you.

It is current practice for a midwife to make the incision but for a doctor to stitch it up, although suturing episiotomies is becoming part of midwifery training and will probably become their routine practice. The stitching needs to be done carefully and some women feel that medical students may not be the best people to do it.

Some midwives feel it reflects on their competence if they allow the vagina to tear in the course of a normal delivery and for this reason may err on safety's side and make an episiotomy when perhaps no action is necessary. This may change as it becomes more usual for midwives to repair episiotomies. An experienced and confident midwife can often help to avoid an episiotomy by her careful handling of the second stage of labour. Her skill and your trust in her can make an enormous difference.

Making yourself more comfortable If you have an episiotomy and sitting or lying feels like you are perched on barbed wire, there are various things you can do. The hospital may offer infra-red or ultrasound treatment to help the healing. You can also:

1 Soak often in a warm bath with salt added; it's a good rest and very soothing.
2 Apply comfrey ointment to the sore places (comfrey ointment or cream is available from some chemists and most health-food shops).
3 Use a child's swimming ring to make sitting more comfortable.
4 The stitches heal better if kept dry – easier said than done. One suggestion is to use a hairdryer (gently!) after going to the loo.
5 There may also be some bruising after prolonged pushing in the second stage of labour which can add to the discomfort. Try *Arnica* for bruising – available in tablet form from homeopathic chemists and some health shops.

Good advice Although the evidence suggests that its routine use is unnecessary, a timely episiotomy can shorten the second stage of labour and avoid the need for a forceps delivery if mother and baby are showing signs of exhaustion or distress. Good advice from the midwife is very useful because pushing *too* hard can increase the risk of a tear or the need for an episiotomy. On the other hand, too much advice from too many people can be confusing: Janet:

> The sensation of the baby's actual birth is something I still relive with astonished delight. The only problem was that besides the midwives I had the Nursing Officer and a trainee GP all trying to deliver me and all shouting at once and telling me not to grunt (!) so when they told me to stop pushing I'd stopped listening and didn't hear them till John repeated it, by which time it was too late and I had a lovely big tear which is still uncomfortable at times.

Many women find the stitching and the after-effects of an episiotomy one of the most distressing aspects of giving birth. It is a procedure that needs a great deal more study and a more sensitive approach from the hospital staff in some cases. Maureen: 'I shall never forget the horror I felt when next morning a staff nurse came to carry out a routine inspection of stitches. On seeing my 'unkindest cut' she yelled at the top of her voice, "Sister, everybody, come and look at this!" I felt like a piece of wet fish on a slab.'

Post-partum haemorrhage (PPH)

Excessive bleeding after the delivery of the baby is probably not more common as a result of increased maternal age, although it may appear so as the incidence does increase with the number of babies a woman has. It is also more common following either unusually rapid or very prolonged labours and is more likely to occur in women who are already anemic. It is to avoid this complication that the delivery of the placenta is usually accelerated by giving an injection of synthetic hormones to contract the uterus after the delivery of the baby.

After this sort of bleeding a blood transfusion may be necessary, but as soon as that is over (it takes about 12 hours) you should feel fine. As I know from my own experience, it doesn't stop you from breastfeeding, although you need a bit of help positioning the baby.

Stillbirth

A very rare possibility, which nevertheless needs to be considered, is that there will not be a live baby at the end of labour – that it will be stillborn. The fact that the baby has died is sometimes known before labour starts because a fetal heart beat cannot be heard. A woman in that position might feel resentful that she has to go through labour knowing the dreadful outcome. However, a Caesarean section would not normally be advised because it is a major operation with possible complications and it is almost always performed on one person for the sake of another – the baby. It is also believed by some that adjustment to the death can be easier if the woman has been through labour. It is worth saying too that a subsequent pregnancy and birth would probably be much easier because it would not be the same as having a first child.

Understandably, a woman may have difficulty coming to terms with the fact that the baby is no longer there and she may not be sure how to look at herself – to be a mother without a child is a strange and painful experience. She is suddenly cut off from other mothers with children but also from women without any. If the couple can be offered the chance to see and hold their baby and perhaps have a photograph to keep, it may become more real. They do need to mourn the death of their baby, even if they have never known her. Pretending it never happened is not a good idea. The death of a baby in the womb needs to be mourned just as any death would be.

Pregnant woman all live to a certain extent with the fear that their baby may die or be handicapped and, in the very rare eventuality of this happening, it can be helpful to share feelings with other people who have had a similar experience (see address list on p. 212 for organizations which could help).

After the Birth

The few days straight after the birth are usually lovely. But it can also be a difficult time. There is a curious kind of double-think about the mother as a patient before and after the birth. During pregnancy you may be treated as if you are ill. Once you've given birth, you may actually *feel* ill (or unwell) or at least very unlike yourself but you can find then that you are left to get on with the business of looking after the baby and your own physical discomforts seem to be of little account.

Adjustment

In the first few days you may feel elated and exhilarated – very excited at having your baby there and holding and caring for her. It is a miraculous feeling after such a long wait.

Cathy's baby arrived early and she was home again after a few hours:

> It was very difficult to adjust to the fact that we actually had a baby. Both John and I found it quite extraordinary that she'd arrived. We repeated to each other over and over again: we've really got a baby and she's staying. It was like having a new toy, no one could take her away and we could cuddle her as much as we liked. It was so exciting and permanent.

It is lucky if you feel high at first because the elation carries you through some of the enormous adjustments you have to make, both physiologically and mentally. Your body has undergone a massive change and will take a while to adjust to its non-pregnant state. As your milk comes in, your breasts might feel tender or hot or become engorged. As you start feeding, your nipples may be sore and you might feel a sharp pull as the uterus contracts, especially when the baby first latches on. My toes used to curl! If you have had an episiotomy, the stitched area is likely to be painful or uncomfortable for a few days at least. It is important to avoid getting constipated – fear of the pain of a bowel movement may put you off but laxatives help. If you had to push for a long time in the second stage, you may get haemorrhoids (piles) internally or externally which makes constipation even less desirable.

Any of these physical discomforts taken singly are quite manageable. Add some of them together, along with lack of sleep and a great excitement and it can all be rather trying at times and exhausting. The mental and emotional adjustments can be even greater. You may have a powerful feeling of unreality and unself at the beginning. There is your baby, you look at her beside your bed and say, 'Is she anything to do with me? Did she really come out of me?' The nursing staff may seem to be forcing you do things you don't feel ready to do and you want to go home. But you're also afraid to go home because how will you manage without all the skilled help on hand?

These changes happen to all mothers but it may be that a woman over 30 has clearer notions about what it will all be like. If it is as you expect, that may be a great help in those first days. However, you might also expect too much of yourself and be disappointed that you can't manage as much as you would like; you might feel unusually vulnerable or inadequate or incompetent. It is as well to be prepared for such feelings and to know that they are shared by so many other mothers. That won't help sufficiently but accepting that it is normal may ease the transition from being pregnant to being a mother.

Tiredness

A word about stamina. In addition to the physical effort of labour and the possible loss of sleep around the time of labour, emotional upheaval is very exhausting. Hospitals are not restful places. Their busy, inflexible schedules can make you feel even more tired and so can visitors, especially having to make social chat with lots of them. It may protect you to ration visitors in the first few days at least (get someone to co-ordinate it). Many women breathe a sigh of relief if the hospital has some fathers-only visiting sessions.

It is also very difficult being separated from your partner at the very time you want to be closest. Diane: 'I felt sad that I was not able to get into my own bed with my husband and have my son with me. My baby was whisked away for bathing and I was wheeled back to a little room alone.' It is possible that when you do see your partner there is little privacy and too much business to catch up on so that what should be a time of great intimacy becomes isolating and you find yourselves getting easily irritated with each other.

Breastfeeding

Most older mothers want to breastfeed and there is no doubt that breast milk is best for babies. Breastfeeding for even a short time will give the baby important antibodies and almost certainly will give both you and your baby a huge amount of pleasure too. It can be difficult to establish breastfeeding in the first few days for a variety of reasons and some women feel the help they get is inadequate. As with many other things, hospital policy and practice may not go together. It may be the policy of the hospital to encourage breastfeeding but the individual mother might not get the right sort of help. Rosalind: 'Somehow no one at antenatal classes mentioned that at least half a dozen different people at the hospital all tell you different things with reference to feeding and no one mentions colic or how to cope with it.'

Probably the most important idea to keep in your head is to breastfeed *soon*, as soon as you can after the birth, and to breastfeed *as often as the baby demands*. Some breastfed babies need feeding as often as every hour or two when they are small. Frequent feeding will stimulate your milk supply and get the baby used to sucking. That sounds like a regime that will play havoc with your own sleep but many babies are quite sleepy in the first week or two and don't demand so much. It is worth persevering even if you have problems. Some contributors who found it difficult to breastfeed in hospital got on much better in the more relaxed atmosphere of their own homes and others managed to re-establish breastfeeding at home even after giving up in hospital. (For more detail about feeding, see chapter 6, p. 115).

Contraception

Before you leave the hospital, someone will probably talk to you about what method of contraception you intend to use now. Sex may be pretty irrelevant to your thinking just then, but you will need to decide what to do. Breastfeeding does not offer adequate protection. There is a fuller discussion of suitable contraceptive methods in chapter 2.

Postnatal depression

It is not unusual for some women to feel depressed after having a baby. The physical and emotional changes are so enormous that it is normal for moods to swing quite violently. Even if you feel bright and elated at first you may feel more dispirited as you get more tired or find that the pain or discomfort you were left with lasts longer than you expected. Although it is quite common to feel tearful and miserable around the fourth or fifth day after delivery, as your hormones change, sometimes you can be made to feel that because you are older *you* shouldn't be weepy.

You can feel depressed postnatally without having postnatal illness. There are perfectly good reasons for some reactive depression. Maybe your baby cries more than you expected (you'd be in good company) and you find that upsetting; you feel desperately tired because you aren't getting the amount or quality of sleep you are used to and feel edgy and miserable; you may miss your job and your colleagues; you may have housing or financial problems. You and your partner have a fair bit of adjusting to do. In some ways it can be helpful if there are adverse circumstances on which to blame the depression or to account for it. If you feel guilty because you think you have no *right* to be depressed, that is an added burden you could do without. It is easy to feel that you have the lovely baby you wanted, you have a home and enough money to manage; furthermore, this is the life you planned and looked forward to, so *why* do you feel so low? And the guilt makes you feel worse.

Expectations A great deal depends on expectations – both your expectations before the birth of what it was going to be like to have a baby, and your expectations of what a good mother should be. A woman over 30 may well have very clear expectations about these things, which differ quite radically from the reality. There is some evidence to suggest that a woman who is 'over the moon' about being pregnant but who doesn't really think about possible changes or adjustments may be slightly more prone to postnatal depression once the reality permeates. Becoming a mother means getting used to a new way of seeing yourself as a woman and this is more difficult and painful for some women than others.

Support Good support is absolutely crucial for a woman who is depressed and also essential to fend off depression. It is more likely to come from other women – mothers, sisters, friends, neighbours, even strangers like a health visitor or postnatal support group. It is very important to be able to talk about how you are feeling, to test out your feelings of uncertainty and inadequacy on someone who can say, 'Yes, I know what it's like. I used to feel like that too.' What you need is sympathetic support and practical help if it can be arranged – like someone taking the baby out for a walk so that you can have a rest or read a book, just have a break to be alone and feel like your old self. What doesn't help is the semi-malicious complacency that goes with comments like 'Oh, just you wait until she starts teething/crawling/walking . . . it will all get much worse.' What you need to be told time and time again as a new mother is that it all gets better because you get better at it and the baby changes as she grows up.

If the depression continues and you are struggling to get through each day, it might be helpful to talk to your doctor. Many women feel a resistance to taking drugs but a short course of anti-depressants or a week or two of sleeping pills might just see you over that particular hump.

Postnatal illness About 10 per cent of mothers, regardless of age, suffer from postnatal depression that is serious enough to be treated as an illness. In its worst and rarest form, 'puerperal psychosis' will probably need hospital treatment. It can be difficult to recognize the signs of postnatal depression and it can start several months after the birth. The most noticeable symptoms are feeling very tired, miserable and irritable and unable to cope with anything. A woman with postnatal depression will crave sleep but often have difficulty sleeping. She will eat more and gain weight which probably makes her feel still worse. Her best time of day might be the morning but by evening she feels very low and tearful. There are various forms of treatment for postnatal depression, often involving a group of tricyclic anti-depressants.

There is a school of thought that believes that low progesterone levels cause postnatal depression and that it can be treated by injections of progesterone. This theory, expressed notably by Dr Katharina Dalton,[2] believes that hormonal changes are crucial in postnatal depression. On the other hand, it may be more helpful to see postnatal depression as a *human* reaction to change. In an article on *Confinement and Depression*, Ann Oakley said, 'Women get depressed after childbirth because in one way and another childbirth and motherhood turn out to be a shock for which they were inadequately prepared.'[3] It has also been suggested that the experience a woman has in hospital around the time of the birth can play a part in whether postnatal depression develops. If the woman feels unhappy about how her labour was managed and particularly if she has not felt free to express this unhappiness; if she finds the staff unhelpful and unsympathetic but puts up with it silently, the suggestion is that she may be more likely to become depressed. An additional factor is thought to be lack of support from her partner or relatives.

When Karen wrote to me about her depression, her baby was nine months old. She was just beginning to feel a little better and found it helpful to write about her experiences. Her story is included in some detail because although there were some unusual circumstances, many of the feelings she describes are shared by other women who have had postnatal depression and the vividness and detail with which she writes makes it all understandable. Her husband was working in Africa when her baby was born in Scotland, and did not arrive in time for the birth.

As the membranes had been leaking fluid, I was advised to report to the hospital for observation 11 days before the baby was due. I was initially admitted for 48 hours which is a rotten way to start as I felt a proper fraud being in hospital when labour hadn't actually started. The staff seemed a bit disinterested and I felt a bit guilty.

The next day the membranes ruptured in the shower, though the staff didn't seem to believe me as the 'evidence' had disappeared down the drain. The antenatal staff in the hospital had built up a feeling of trust and teamwork and the actual stay in hospital was very disappointing as everyone seemed so busy and there was no meaningful communication. By 10.30 a.m. I was shaved, no enema, and half sitting, half lying on a narrow, hard delivery bed in a windowless boring room. I really could have done with my husband's company for moral support as I felt quite overpowered by the institution. I felt that everyone was very busy and didn't have time to talk to me or indeed even expect me to want to ask any questions. By 12 noon I was attached to a drip of glucose and Syntocinon. I was mainly on my own till after 4.30 p.m., the odd head popping round the door to ask if I was OK or to turn up the drip. I wasn't really OK as I was lonely, tired, bored, and uncomfortable from half sitting on backache. At about 5 p.m. someone asked me if I could feel contractions which they could feel by touching my abdomen. I am only guessing now but imagine I was given pethidine not long after that. I wasn't asked if I wanted drugs or told that I'd been given any but I was drowsy from then on.

It must have been about 7.45 p.m. when I felt the urge to start pushing. My morale was low and I began to worry that all was not well with the baby. When the second stage of labour got going the baby felt stuck. I could feel him jammed up against me inside. The midwives were trying really hard to encourage me. 'Come on now, Mrs White, if you want your baby delivered tonight.' I felt I was being criticized for my poor efforts. 'Chin down and push.' I longed to throw off that damned drip, grab hold of something solid in each hand, brace my feet against the wall and *push*. Now the nurses told me they could see the baby's head at the height of each contraction. 'Try a bit harder', they said! I couldn't try any harder. 'He's stuck', I thought, 'He's jammed up against my insides.' I was convinced the baby was dying. The doctor did a low forceps delivery and held him up – very blue and silent and still.

He was born at 8.34 p.m. and about ten minutes later he was brought briefly back to me to hold. I hardly felt he was mine. The doctors had delivered him, breathed life into him. He looked so battered and bruised. 'Poor thing', I thought, 'you've had a rough time and your daddy isn't here.' The baby spent his first three days in special care and I could only see him at daytime feeds, after the SCBU staff 'phoned my ward to 'invite' me. No one suggested that I might want to go and just look at him.

Breastfeeding was difficult. I have inverted nipples. The baby cried frantically and couldn't fix on to my folding nipples. The SCBU was hot. My tail end was really sore. The student midwives in the SCBU looked as though they thought I was stupid trying to breastfeed with so much trouble.

I felt clumsy and inadequate. Old and useless. Most of the other mums were younger than me. I felt they thought I was a stupid old fusspot (they probably didn't even notice me). Always they said at night, 'We'll just take him down to the nursery' and I felt I couldn't say no. He was disturbing other people. He was hospital property, not mine. I lay awake. I dozed, dreamed he had died and woke up really believing it. I lay awake and cried.

By the time I left hospital I was already on the road to depression. I was riddled with guilt and worry, my confidence was smashed. (Logic: you've failed the baby at birth and feeding, what else will you fail him in?) I was physically below par, full of aches and pains, and utterly tired but unable to sleep or even rest well and I had effectively cut myself off from any lifeline, any safety valve. I felt no one would understand, that I had to tackle it all alone.

Karen continued to face it alone for months even after she joined her husband in Africa weeks later. Finally, in desperation, she wrote to the Association for Postnatal Illness (see p. 212 for the address).

> It helped put everything in perspective. It opened the floodgates of meaningful discussion with my husband. I could turn to him and say, 'This is how I feel.' I could show him that other people had felt this way – that I really couldn't help the lethargy, the self-pity, pessimism, irritability, etc.

Karen found it easier then to talk to other people and found it helped. She went back to Scotland and to the maternity hospital where her baby was born and asked questions about the birth. She found out by chance that her baby was born with the umbilical cord tightly round his neck and that made her feel better about the blame she had attached to herself. After nine months she was beginning to feel more like herself and more optimistic about the future.

Attitudes of hospital staff Many of the things that happened to Karen were dreadfully unfortunate and make it easy to see why she became depressed. However, a very important factor in what happened to her was the way she perceived the attitudes of the hospital staff. The lack of real interest in her as a person was vitally important to her at a difficult time.

Many of my volunteers had experiences which suggested that the hospital staff simply didn't listen to them. A number of women were not believed when they said they were in labour. One was told she was constipated, given lunch on the antenatal ward and when she vomited, was given an injection because she was 'hysterical'. Her baby was born three hours later and her husband missed the birth because he had been sent home. Another woman, who was also not believed to be in labour was found shortly afterwards to be 'sitting on the baby's head'.

Many women justifiably feel that if hospital staff paid more attention to them as people who might be in touch with what was happening to their bodies and talked to them rather than about them, their births would have been happier occasions. Lack of continuity of midwife care during labour was a frequently mentioned drawback. Maggie: 'The only problem with my labour was the change of midwives halfway through due to a change of shift. I did not like the second midwife. The first was informative and helpful.' Those women who were lucky enough to have the same midwife throughout labour and delivery were appreciative of the support and the more personal attention they received.

Joyful labour

Pauline describes her experience like this:

> When my waters broke it was like waking on the morning of a very important exam for which I'd done an immense amount of work – a feeling of excitement anticipation that here was what I had been training for. I think I kept fairly calm and didn't have to have any painkillers. My main memory is of overwhelming pressure, of my whole body being taken over by this tiny thing struggling out, and of looking up to see the wet, limp little creature lying helplessly on my thighs and later, of

seeing her tiny face peeping out of a towel having her first meal.

I loved breastfeeding her – it seemed miraculous that I could keep her alive like that.

After hearing about Pauline's antenatal experiences on p. 43, it is worth pausing to remember that giving birth is one of the most marvellous and exciting experiences of your life. If there is pain, it isn't like other pain. For one thing, you know the reason for it and that it won't go on for ever. For another, and quite unlike other pain, it has a purpose – there is a wonderfully creative outcome at the end of it all. Another reassuring aspect is that you are not alone – you have the support and sympathy and expertise of midwives who can help you through even frightening or uncomfortable stages. The trust you have that your midwife is working with you and wants to see the baby born before she goes off duty, makes it feel as if you are really sharing it. Then it is all over and you are face to face with the baby who has grown inside you. Angela:

> I looked carefully into my newborn's face. She was neither raw-red nor wrinkled. Her cheeks were pink and firm, like little well-set jellies. Her nose was tip-tilted and minute. What intrigued me most was her attitude. She lounged in my arms like a pampered female maharajah, eyes loosely-lidded, hands folded lightly over her chest. She looked a trifle bored – somewhat disdainful. She seemed to be watching some dull court pageant and was clearly not amused. The name Victoria was going to suit this infant beautifully.
>
> She suddenly decided to have some refreshment and started rooting for the breast. She clamped her jaws on me hungrily and chomped away with zest. My husband and I laughed together in joy. Victoria was a survivor and she knew her business. As she fed, I looked at her tiny feet in wonderment. They were exquisite – neat and dainty as a doll's. Her hands were tiny too, spread out like pink baby starfishes. How had my husband and I, such heavy, big-boned people, managed to produce such a feminine-looking little girl? She weighed a robust 9 lbs but it felt like less.

Labour and the immediate postnatal period will vary greatly for each woman. Like everybody else, you would like to go through your pregnancy and labour as normally as possible and if you have prepared yourself for natural childbirth you may feel strongly that you do not wish to have much medical intervention in labour. As long as labour progresses normally this should be possible but it may be longer or more difficult than anticipated. Any interventions that are recommended, including the use of pain-killing drugs, need to be considered in the light of your own wishes and circumstances. The delivery bed is not the best place to fight a battle so it is worth working out beforehand what kind of birth you would like and making sure that these points are clearly visible in your notes. To be realistic, you should also think about what you would like if everything isn't completely straightforward. Hopefully then you will feel as Helen did: 'It was hard work but the most tremendous experience and a fantastic feeling of achievement.'

5

The Risk to the Baby

It is quite natural for every pregnant woman to wonder whether her baby will be normal and healthy. A woman over 30 also has to face the slightly greater risk of having a handicapped child. However, you can be made unnecessarily anxious during pregnancy by the vagueness of the stories you hear about maternal age and abnormality. One woman told me that the worry was always there, gnawing away at her and haunting her dreams throughout her pregnancy.

There is no question that Down's syndrome (mongolism) and certain other disorders which involve chromosomal abnormality become more common with the mother's increasing age. However, there is no evidence to suggest that an older first-time mother has a greater chance of producing a baby which has other congenital defects, merely because of her age. Statistically, all first babies are at greater risk than the second or third child born to each woman – the functioning of the uterus improves with some practice. The risks increase again with the fifth and subsequent babies.

Perinatal and neonatal mortality

It is very difficult to assess the health and wellbeing of newborn babies in statistical form. For this reason, the rather crude measure of the number of babies who *fail* to survive early life is used when assessing the problems that still face the mother and baby and as an index of the progress in providing better care for them. Two figures are used. The *perinatal mortality rate* includes all babies who die *in utero* once the pregnancy is more than 28 weeks and all babies who die within the first week of birth. The *neonatal mortality rate* includes all babies who die within four weeks of birth.

There are several major problems that contribute to perinatal mortality. These include babies born with serious abnormalities, babies born very prematurely and those who suffer deprivation of oxygen in pregnancy or in labour. There has been concern for some time that the perinatal and neonatal mortality rates in Britain are too high, much higher than in many other industrialized countries. Furthermore, they are improving more slowly than in many poorer countries. A parliamentary committee under the chairmanship of Renée Short that enquired into this area in 1979–80 suggested that between a third and a half of perinatal and neonatal deaths are preventable. The report pinpointed many avoidable factors but as yet very few of its recommendations have been implemented. Some would be extremely expensive in manpower and equipment but some of the simpler recommendations include better immunization programmes against rubella (German measles), a greater realization of the damage done by smoking and an improvement in diet, especially among young, unsupported mothers and some immigrant groups who have an inadequate diet for cultural reasons. The report isolates two types of predisposing factors involved in perinatal mortality:

1 *biological factors* such as congenital deformity or the presence of hereditary disorders in the parents, which require diagnosis before conception and treatment or genetic counselling;
2 *environmentally or socio-economically determined risks*: poor nutrition, physique, chronic infection, poor pregnancy spacing or unplanned pregnancy often at the extremes of parental age; ignorance of the benefits to be gained from good medical care.[1]

There is virtually no other reference in the report to maternal age except as a risk factor in relation to Down's syndrome.

It is important to state here that many current figures about maternal age and risks to the baby are not very helpful to the new group of older first-time mothers who have planned and prepared for their pregnancies. As we have already said, many of these women are in the upper socio-economic groups. There is a strong link between perinatal and neonatal mortality and many birth defects and social class – the higher the social class, the lower the risk.[2]

This effect overrides the increase in risk with rising maternal age. The British Births Survey of 1970 studied every birth in England, Scotland and Wales during one week in April 1970. There was a high perinatal mortality rate in very young mothers and in mothers over 35.[3] However, many of the mothers in the older age-group then suffered the disadvantages mentioned in the Short Report, especially those of rapid, unplanned pregnancy (some of them had five children or more) and chronic nutritional problems. The group of women now having their first babies in their thirties and forties are usually highly motivated to look after themselves well during pregnancy and are less likely to be either very poor or malnourished.

Serious birth defects

About one in 40 babies has some birth defect, the majority being very minor and unlikely to interfere with a normal healthy life. For example, my son Ben was born with six fingers on each hand, something I had never heard of but now know is a well-recognized occurrence. It is quite difficult to remember that they were ever there – the extra fingers were tied off in the first week after birth and there remain only minute scars that he'll be able to boast about later on.

The majority of birth defects occur by chance. A few are clearly hereditary and some have well-known associations. Of severe defects, 3–5 per cent are thought to be the result of some chromosomal abnormality and these are related to the age of the mother (and in a few cases to the age of the father). The relationship of maternal age to birth defects that are *not* chromosomal is statistically insignificant.[4] For some defects, an older mother is at no disadvantage. For example, the incidence of spina bifida and other neural tube defects is related to geographical area rather than age – being most common in Scotland, Ireland and South Wales.[5] Spina bifida can be detected after a screening test for alpha-fetoprotein (see p. 46), but this is not used routinely in all areas.

A study of congenital postural deformities at Birmingham Maternity Hospital in 1960–1 carried out by Dr Peter Dunn showed that there was no substantial difference in the number of deformed infants born to women over 30.[6] The study covered a wide range of deformities that had arisen in later fetal life altering the form or structure of a previously formed part, like dislocation of the hip or positional abnormality of the feet. Many of these are minor abnormalities which can be corrected easily after birth. In a later paper on postural deformities Dr Dunn offers a salutory reminder: 'The price paid for a larger and more mature infant at birth, better able to stand the pressures of extrauterine life, is a 2 per cent incidence of deformities. Perhaps we ought rather to marvel at the fact that 98 per cent of infants are *not* deformed at birth and that 90 per cent of those that are will correct spontaneously after birth.'[7]

Chromosomal defects

The well-known danger to an older first-time mother, and one that increases as she gets older, is of chromosomal abnormality leading, in particular, to Down's syndrome.

Chromosomes are collections of genes. Each cell in the body contains 46 of these rod-like chromosomes, arranged in pairs. The character of the gene dictates our development from the moment of conception and the addition of the smallest piece of this material has a profound effect on fetal development. In order to ensure that the correct gene balance is maintained at fertilization, sperms and ova contain only 23 chromosomes, one from each pair.

There are various *known causes* of chromosomal abnormality:

1 excessive X-ray exposure before or during pregnancy;
2 exposure of either parent to certain chemicals (as happened in Seveso in Italy in 1974);
3 some virus infections;
4 some hereditary diseases.

Most important for the purpose of this book are those of *advancing maternal age* or, more rarely, advanced paternal age. Most chromosomal abnormalities are incompatible with life and the fetus is spontaneously aborted. The small proportion that do survive tend to be the less severe cases, e.g. Turner's syndrome, a sex chromosomal abnormality where one X chromosome is missing, producing defects compatible with life. Nevertheless, 95 per cent of fetuses with Turner's syndrome abort in the first three months.

Down's syndrome Down's syndrome (or mongolism) was discovered in 1959 to be a chromosomal abnormality in which some cells contain *an extra chromosome*, giving a total of 47 c. It is now known that the extra chromosome belongs to pair No. 21 and is technically known as trisomy 21. This particular abnormality accounts for about half the babies born with disorders of chromosome numbers as we presently understand them. The others include several rare trisomies and a number of conditions in which there is an incorrect number of sex chromosomes. The trisomy of Down's syndrome can occur in two ways, by processes called translocation and non-disjunction, only the latter being connected with maternal age.

Translocation occurs when, in the cells of either parent, a chromosome of the 21 pair becomes stuck to a chromosome of another pair, usually No. 15. The total number of chromosomes present in the parent cell is normal and the possessor of the anomaly is normal. This state is known as being the carrier of a balanced translocation. Unfortunately, it is possible that when ova or sperms are formed, the hitchhiking No. 21 chromosome may pass into these cells with the free No. 21 and on fertilization the developing fetus will contain an extra set of the genetic information carried on the 21 chromosome, and will have Down's syndrome. This accounts for a small proportion of children with this syndrome and is independent of parental age. If there is a history of mongolism in the family of one or other parent, a blood test can be performed to ascertain whether he or she is a carrier. Carriers of a balanced translocation are capable of producing children with normal chromosomes. If such an abnormality is found you should discuss the probable outcome of future pregnancies with an expert geneticist.

Table 1 shows the incidence of Down's syndrome in relation to maternal age. The overall incidence of Down's syndrome for all ages is 1.67 per thousand births in the British population.[8] Tables that cover a range of ages can, however, be misleading for a specific age – the information is more reliable seen as a graph (see Figure 1). Whichever way the figures are presented, the incidence of this condition increases with maternal age.

Down's syndrome, in common with the other disorders of chromosome number, produces a characteristic appearance in affected children. They have a flattened back to their heads, a flat face, a protruding tongue, low-set ears, a short neck and stubby fingers. (A word of warning – many newborn babies may initially have slightly odd-shaped heads because of the natural changes which occur in labour. These go away in a few days and are *not* evidence of Down's syndrome.) In addition to their characteristic appearance they are all mentally retarded but their level of intelligence varies considerably. They also have a higher than usual incidence of heart defects, intestinal abnormalities, eye and ear problems.

Table 1

Maternal age	Incidence of Down's syndrome per 1,000 births
15–19	0.54
20–24	0.63
25–29	0.75
30–34	1.23
35–39	3.82
40–44	10.72
45+	18.63

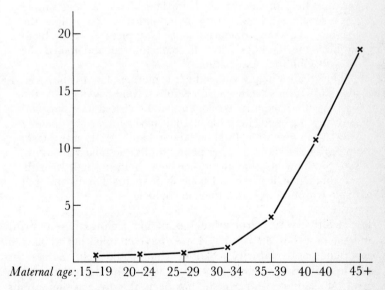

Figure 1 Incidence of Down's Syndrome per 1,000 births

There is increasing new evidence to suggest that many of these children are capable of much more than was previously thought possible. With patient teaching, many can learn to cope with the simpler tasks of everyday living. Others have been taught to read and write and operate with a surprising degree of independence. One Down's syndrome young woman recently won a Duke of Edinburgh Gold Award and has a part-time job in a canteen. There seems to be untapped potential in some of these children. They also tend to be very equable, placid and loving. There is a parental support organization for parents of Down's children (see p. 213 for the address).

Carol, who first contacted me after she had her first baby at 31, then had another baby who has Down's syndrome. Kate was seven months old when Carol wrote again:

> It was ironic for me as, being a nurse and a midwife, I had often dwelt on the possibility of handicap and had decided that I could accept treatable conditions but mental handicap would be very hard. When Kate was born I wished she could have had a heart defect instead as I had nursed so many children following complex surgery and watched them recover. However, we immediately contacted all the agencies that could possibly help or inform us. Kate herself was a help simply because she is a lovable little baby and it is easy to love the lovable. We read copiously, looked at pictures, read biographies, met families with affected children and joined the Down's Children Association.
>
> The greatest help was meeting the mother of a little boy who also had Down's syndrome, on Kate's second day of life. At the request of a paediatric social worker she visited us in hospital with my husband there too. I shall never forget her opening words: 'So you want to know about Paul?' With enthusiasm and pride she showed us her photographs and talked about her son. She now also has two other boys, both normal. It made me think that if she could cope with such a family and still bounce around in jeans, then so could I.

The positive way Carol writes about her feelings is reassuring and the fact that she is now 34 may have enabled her to use her experience and maturity to know what would help them – the information they needed, how to go about finding it and who to turn to for advice. In turn, she has been able to visit the parents of another mongol baby through her local NCT group.

Although the proportion of mongols is thought to be about the same as it used to be, seven or eight times as many mongol children reach school age compared with the 1920s because of better medical care.[9] (People with Down's syndrome often don't live after the age of 20, although with a milder form of the condition this can be considerably extended.) It is possible to detect Down's syndrome antenatally (see p. 48) and a pregnant woman carrying a Down's syndrome fetus will be offered a termination if she wishes. The risks of these procedures, notably of amniocentesis in terms of spontaneous abortion or fetal damage, are discussed on p. 49.

Preterm babies

A baby is considered to be preterm if born earlier than 37 weeks gestation. This concept replaces the old idea that a baby was premature if she weighed less than 2.5 kg at birth. A preterm baby is at risk of developing problems after birth because her body is immature and not yet fully prepared for the extrauterine environment. Under these circumstances the baby may need the facilities and expertise of special neonatal units. The main problems that arise are those of temperature control and breathing difficulties where the baby's lungs are inelastic and cannot take in sufficient air. Feeding may also be difficult as the sucking reflex may not have developed and these young babies have great difficulty maintaining their body temperature. To be cared for as safely as possible, the baby usually spends her first few days in an incubator surrounded by what seems a formidable array of machinery. Most of these are there simply to watch and warn if the baby shows signs of developing problems.

Special-care Baby Units may appear frightening and remote places and sometimes the staff in them seem so wrapped up in their intensive care of the babies in them that parents feel there is little place for them. Watching one's baby weather these early problems in a strange environment when so tiny and vulnerable is frightening and unreal. It's difficult to believe she could ever survive. The staff of a good Special-Care Unit realize the worries that parents face and do their best to explain what is happening, make visiting the baby as free as possible and encourage parents to do as much caring for the baby as circumstances permit. You should also get advice and help in getting the supply of breast milk established so that your milk can be given to the baby and, when she is old enough to suck normally, she will be able to breastfeed normally.

There are several identified reasons for preterm labours. It is known that heavy smokers are more likely to delivery before 37 weeks of pregnancy and that those in lower socio-economic groups carry a greater risk. The risk increases with each pregnancy after the fourth and there is an association with poor weight gain in pregnancy. The 1958 birth survey revealed that women over the age of 35 had a greater chance of preterm births at 37 weeks.[10] However, most of those women were what is called 'grand multips', i.e. they had had five or more children. A study in 1976 showed no increase in spontaneous preterm births with increasing maternal age.[11]

Intrauterine deprivation

The final large group of disadvantaged babies are those who suffer lack of nutrition or oxygen *in utero*, either during pregnancy or in labour. In its chronic form, this results in the baby growing poorly and being born smaller than expected. These 'light-for-dates' babies have poor energy reserves in the first days of life and may become cold or develop hypoglycaemia (low blood–sugar levels). If the intrauterine starvation is severe it can result in poor development of the baby and leave permanent problems, occasionally even leading to a stillbirth. Fortunately, the majority of these babies rapidly make up for lost time and soon regain their expected weight after birth. There are many reasons for intrauterine growth retardation. Some are totally unexplained but in many instances light-for-dates babies are born to women who are heavy smokers or who have underlying medical problems such as hypertension (see p. 57).

The older first-time mother does carry a slightly increased risk of producing a small baby because she is more likely to suffer from a predisposing medical problem. However, in fit women the risk is very small.

Conclusion

When contemplating a pregnancy, a woman over 30 has little special reason to fear that she will have an abnormal baby. One in 40–50 babies has a defect at birth, usually tiny and correctible, regardless of the age of the mother. There is a definite and increasing risk of Down's syndrome with maternal age and it is probably advisable to seek an amniocentesis after the age of 38 or 39. It is also important to realize that even at the upper end of the reproductive age range at 45, the risk of Down's syndrome is only about 2 per cent. The statistics may offer some reassurance but can only give an overview and are no comfort to those individuals who do have to face the difficult and painful experience of the birth of a handicapped child.

This chapter aims to place the risks to the baby of an older mother in some sort of overall perspective which suggests that apart from the dramatic link of chromosomal abnormality with maternal age, advancing maternal age alone does not increase the risk to the baby. The general health of the mother, her approach to her pregnancy in terms of issues like nutrition, smoking, antenatal care, her social class and circumstances are all more significant than her age in possible risks to her infant.

6

The First Six Weeks or So

Aleid is Dutch. When she was 38, she had married a British man, moved to Manchester to live in a house with five other adults and started a new job, all within a week. Then a year later she had a baby. After living alone for nine years, and working and studying in Holland, the changes were immense.

> The first few weeks I thought that if other people suffer from postnatal depression, then I definitely had postnatal exhilaration. I felt on top of the world all the time. It was quite constant, a basic feeling of great happiness. I also cried a lot but it wasn't out of sadness – it was just because it was all so *much*. It had to go somewhere so I cried. It lasted a long time – months. I felt absolutely *great*.

She goes on:

> I still feel that it's *lovely* not to work, to stay at home and look after him and be quiet and recover from all the changes.

Aleid had been closely involved with her sister's two children from the start.

> She brought them up in a way that I thought was really nice and I think that in what I'm doing now, I've had a good example. It makes me more secure.

It isn't like that for everybody. Anna had little experience of other people's babies and was living in a flat in London with her partner when she had her first baby at 34.

> I was expecting tiredness, deflation, anxiety, etc, but didn't realize how demanding a newborn baby is and how depressed and pessimistic and drained I would feel. Everyone kept saying what a lovely baby he was, but for the first two to three weeks, until he started smiling and responding and not crying every instant he wasn't asleep or feeding, I couldn't have cared how lovely he was or wasn't. I would have welcomed somebody around who could sympathize and accept how I was feeling and yet who could also say (convincingly), 'It will get better soon, you will love your baby and he'll love you and you'll enjoy it. Just hang on for the first six weeks.'

You may not feel like either Aleid or Anna but their experiences show that there are very different ways of reacting to the birth of your baby and there is no way of knowing how *you* are going to feel until it happens to you. It will depend on the sort of birth you had and its after-effects; how much help you have at home; how relaxed and confident you feel; your partner's approach; how settled and easy the baby is; how well the feeding goes. If you feel more like Anna, try to give yourelf the encouragement she would have liked to hear: just hang on for the first six weeks.

Why six weeks?

Six weeks isn't a magic time. In spite of what other people tell you, your baby's feeding might not have settled into a routine by then; she might not be cutting out a night feed yet. In fact, if she's breastfed she might not cut out all night feeds for a year or so. The only thing you can be sure will happen at six weeks is that you'll be given a postnatal check-up (and probably be signed off) and so will your baby. But the first few weeks (whether for you it happens to be four, six or eight) are an important settling down time – for your body, for you and your baby, for the other people you live with. If you live with a partner, both of you will now have to adjust to being not two but three. After those weeks have passed you will gradually see yourself in a much more relaxed phase: you won't be anxious about doing the right thing, you'll feel better physically, you will have worked out the most convenient way of arranging things – a milestone will have been reached.

Milestones happen all the time with babies. You will almost certainly mark the first smile, the first tooth, the first crawl, the first babble, the first night she sleeps right through and you wake up in a sweat thinking something awful has happened because she hasn't cried. You will also forget most of those things quite quickly. Try asking someone else who has a child older than yours about one of the practical details that absorb you. As often as not, she'll say she can't remember. There are so many stages and it seems that before you're out of one, you're into the next. But until you get used to this rapid change and development, be easy on yourself. Expect some confusion, some questioning, some swings of mood and unique tiredness as well as indescribable happiness. Rita: 'I can't remember finding anything difficult. I was in a state of euphoria for weeks. I felt reborn myself – experiencing sights and sounds as if for the first time.'

Settling in at home

Since you are likely to have your baby in hospital, you will certainly feel pleased when you can go home. Few people enjoy being in hospital and you may find it a less than ideal place in which to get to know your baby. It is also hard to have to see your partner only when it suits the hospital. You might miss the closeness and relaxation of home; there is bound to be too much to talk about and he will want to get to know the baby too. It is a good idea to involve your partner early on and let him do things for the baby – wash, dress, change, hold and cuddle her even if she is asleep.

In spite of all the good things about going home you might also feel a bit anxious and insecure, since the advice and help that was on hand in the maternity ward won't be so readily available. There will be no nursery where you can take the baby if she is restless or you want to have a bath; meals might well not be put in front of you three times a day.

All hospitals seem to operate at hothouse temperatures but when you get home you don't have to keep your whole house at 80°F. The room where the baby sleeps and where she spends her day should be about 68°F and, when you bath her, she should be kept warm too. You will probably have decided where you want the baby to sleep before you go home, even if those ideas changed when you confronted the snuffling, snorting reality of your baby. I found that I was so twitchy about every tiny sound my baby made that it was better for my own sleep to have him in another room. Lynne didn't find that for long:

> With the night feeds, as soon as I put Matthew down in his cot he was awake again. The inevitable happened. One night I was lying in bed feeding him, and the next thing I had fallen fast asleep and knew nothing until morning. It was the first decent amount of sleep I had had since he was born. After that he slept with us every night until he was ten months when he was quite happy to sleep through and has never been a problem in that way since. The first few nights Richard and I ended up huddled on the far end of the bed because we were so frightened of suffocating Matthew. Then we realized that he was actually extremely mobile in bed because the soft sheets supported the weight of his head and that early crawling reflex actually has a purpose! He never fell out of bed because he always moved towards the warmth. He actually like snuggling up so close to me that my breasts almost seemed to suffocate him. Has there ever been a real case of a baby suffocating in bed with his (sober) parents I wonder?

It's a good point. You don't need to worry about rolling on top of your baby in bed – it is extremely unlikely and anyway, she'd cry if you did. Apart from her sleeping place, it is worth giving some thought to where you are going to keep all the paraphernalia of changing and dressing her – the nappies, clothes, plastic pants, cotton wool, zinc and castor oil cream, etc. It is probably most convenient to keep all these things in one place but it need not be a cold upstairs bedroom. Some women I know use the living room because that is where they spend most of their time and it is warm. If you have backache it can help to use a table or chest of drawers for changing, or to kneel beside a bed, anywhere that means you can avoid bending. But do be careful. Even though most babies don't start rolling around on their own before 3–4 months, yours may be the energetic exception and floors are very hard.

Don't expect too much of yourself You will need time to be alone with the people you live with – whether it is one partner or several people in the household – and to spend time together with the baby. Ask your friends to phone if that's possible before they come to visit, otherwise you could be inundated. Don't be afraid to ask someone to call again another time if you're feeding or bathing the baby and would be happier to be doing that without having to chat to someone at the same time. Pinning a note on the door saying you're having a rest, or taking the phone off the hook are perfectly reasonable self-protective measures. And you do need to protect yourself.

Get some help If you live with other people you should be able to get by doing very little other than looking after yourself and the baby for a while. Aleid found that living in a house with four other adults made a huge difference – after a while she really wanted to be allowed to cook! If you live with a man he will be able to do some of the housework but what he does and how much will depend on how used he is to doing it, how he sees his best efforts being spent now and how he is adjusting to the new and strange feelings of being a father.

A relative or friend might offer help. Be honest about whether you want it. If it means the person staying with you, be aware that that may create extra difficulties rather than lighten yours. One woman whose mother came to stay for a fortnight ended up looking after the baby *and* her mother.

The midwife will call every day for the first two weeks and after that a health visitor will call regularly. They won't usually offer practical help (although the midwife might bath the baby once or twice) but can be helpful and reassuring when it comes to answering questions. Write down any queries as they occur to you otherwise they are bound to vanish when the midwife calls. Whatever time she does call you can be sure it will be when you are in the bath or in the middle of a feed or talking on the phone – that's the way of these things.

You might be able to get a *home help*. It is a statutory right that a woman should be entitled to home help for two weeks after having a baby but the cutbacks in social services have made this much more uncommon. If you had a difficult birth and are not well, or if you have little or no help at home, you ought to be able to get some help. You pay a minimum amount but the number of hours' help (between four and twelve) are assessed according to your need. If you are anxious about managing at home talk to the ward sister before you leave the hospital or to your GP or midwife immediately afterwards.

Tiredness

Every new parent includes tiredness as one of the most difficult things to cope with in the early weeks (or even months). At the very time you need sleep most to restore your strength and help you cope with the new demands, it is denied and the loss comes as a shock. Jill Tweedie, writing in *The Guardian* about herself as a very young mother of 18, describes her horror when: 'The nurse informed me that this little stranger would have to be fed every four hours, day and night. I simply didn't believe her. I can't do it in the *night*, I said, reasoning with a mad-woman. I *sleep* in the night you see.'[1] Even people 20 years older might not have absorbed the fact that their sleep would be interrupted. Paul has lots of friends with children and had talked with them before William was born, but

> I expected him to sleep as many hours as I would sleep, at least eight hours continuously. That had never been explained to me. I knew you had to feed them but I thought that straight after feeding and winding he'd go back to sleep. That wasn't the case. There was a whole series of shocks one after the other but I think because you've cleared your mind and were expecting changes, you could cope better.

What Paul is saying here is important because even if he had known more about babies' sleeping patterns, it is almost impossible to 'explain' to someone else exactly how tired you may feel once there is a new baby in the house. The degree of tiredness is probably different from anything you've known before (certainly different from staying up late at night or working very hard or studying intensively) and it is cumulative, building up over a period of time. Everyone says you will be tired but when it happens to you there is still some surprise. So there does seem to be some unavoidable mismatch between hearing from others (who may also be afraid of putting you off) and experiencing it yourself. All the more difficult if you are on your own, like Yvonne:

> I had no idea you could *be* so tired, e.g. one night Sam was sleeping in the bed with me and he fell out. I woke up and heard the thud as he fell on the floor. He didn't make a noise

for a minute and I lay there thinking, 'He's dead. That's all right. I don't have to wake up, there's nothing I can do.' And then he started screaming and I thought, 'Well, that's fine. He's alive.' And I had to *force* myself to wake up to pick him up and put him back in the bed.

Another thing I did once: I used to bath him, put the baby bath in the upstairs bath, bring him down, sit on the floor here in front of the fire, dry him, dress him, feed him off to sleep, put him over my shoulder carrying him back up the stairs to put him face down in his cot in his bedroom. And one night I put him face down in the bath, in the cold water. And I couldn't understand why he'd woken up. Just for a moment I thought, 'But he doesn't wake up when I put him down. He stays asleep.' I was so *befuddled* that I couldn't make the connection between him screaming and the fact that I'd put him in the cold bath water.

Adjusting to the difficulties The experience of lost hours and broken sleep can be quite disturbing although fortunately there don't seem to be any long-term ill effects. The quality of rest may change too – you may sleep very lightly, half-listening in case the baby wakes. That may interfere with the opportunity to dream and it is suggested that dream deprivation affects general wellbeing. During the day you may find it difficult to switch off sufficiently to sleep when the baby does.

It takes time to adjust to the new pattern, to take the chance to catch up on sleep when you can, rather than doing other things. You may be surprised by how absent-minded and forgetful you become for a while after the birth and despair at your normally cool, competent brain's refusal to concentrate. Some of that distractedness may be brought about by constant unexpected interruption to whatever you are doing (and that continues as the baby grows up) but some of it is caused by insufficient sleep and rest. Lack of sleep may also make you irritable and slow down your reactions – significant if you drive.

The perspective of age The advantage your age and experience gives you is being able to reason that even if things are difficult now, it won't last forever. Your baby *will* start sleeping for longer periods and so will you and even if she still wakes up during the night, as many babies do, you will get used to it and settling her will take less and less time. Those initial six weeks might seem long at the time but deep down you *know* that six weeks is nothing, even a year goes by in a flash. A younger person possibly has less of a sense of continuity and of how things move on regardless.

Your body

Your shape and weight Tiredness may not be the only factor in what sometimes feels like a struggle to survive. It can be disappointing to find that you do not lose much more than the baby's weight at first and that you still aren't anywhere near to doing up a skirt. You may feel fat and flabby and it is quite natural to feel put out about that. It can be really hard to get yourself to do the exercises that will help you to get rid of that wobbly flesh. You'll probably be taught postnatal exercises in the hospital but it requires tremendous discipline to fit them into the schedule. It might be a good idea to get together with another woman who has just had a baby and do your exercises together or go to a postnatal exercise class. That has the double advantage of getting you out and giving you a break and getting back into shape. By the end of six weeks you should be getting nearer your pre-pregnant state but you will probably still weigh more and your stretched skin will take more work to tighten up. Swimming helps you do that as well as other exercises.

If you are breastfeeding you will use up an extra 500–1,000 calories a day more than you did when you were pregnant, so it's not a good idea to diet at this stage. You need to be well-nourished to maintain your health, your wellbeing and, so, your milk supply. Losing a lot of weight suddenly mobilizes your fat supplies and your milk may then contain higher levels of potentially dangerous chemicals. What you eat and drink will affect your milk so you need to choose carefully and avoid too much of anything that might upset your baby, particularly a lot of alcohol or high amounts of caffeine in tea and coffee.

Physical discomfort

- If you have had an episiotomy your *stitches may hurt* for a week or two or even longer. On p. 85 there are some suggestions that might help.
- You may get *piles* (haemorrhoids) especially if there was a long second stage of labour with a lot of pushing. It is

important not to get constipated if you have piles, so eat lots of high-fibre foods like whole grains, wholemeal bread and fresh fruit and vegetables. You might need to get suppositories or a cream from your doctor.

● *Wind* is quite common and can add embarrassingly to the feeling of your body not being quite in your control.

● Your *skin* may get spotty or feel itchy or dry.

● Your *nipples may be sore* at first. If so, talk to the midwife.

● Your *back may ache* and may continue to ache because babies are heavy and get heavier; they also need a tremendous amount of carrying and lifting up and down. Try to bend from your knees and to work with your baby (changing, bathing her) at a height that is comfortable for you, e.g. you can bath her in a bowl on a table rather than having to bend over the big bath.

● Your *hair may fall out* a bit but that, though disconcerting, is common and soon stops.

Now for the good news. Not all of this catalogue of disasters is likely to affect *you* – unless you're very unlucky – and you might actually *feel a lot better* after the birth. Lindsay:

> When I was first at home with my baby after my two days in hospital, I felt very light and active. I felt much brighter than when pregnant, more alert mentally and much more sociable. Although I felt very tired at times, because of the inevitable broken nights, I found it much easier to push the pram up the hill on which I live than it had been to walk up it breathlessly when very pregnant. I feel that friends stressed the drawbacks of having a new baby and few people mentioned the rewards that babies give in terms of their warmth and cuddliness.

Some women feel so excited and elated by having a baby that the buzz carries them over the tiredness of the first weeks. It does help if you can get out and about and do some of the things you've always enjoyed. It is really quite easy to take a baby with you to all sorts of places, especially if you are breastfeeding. Many restaurants don't mind a carry-cot; you can take your baby to meetings and films; we took Ben to our local pub when he was three weeks old and left him asleep in the carry-cot on the table. It is also good for other people to see babies and to accept that often they can go where you go. It is surprising what a difference it makes to go out for a bit especially if you've been feeling a bit ground down. It can seem an effort to organize but releases new energy so it's worth taking the trouble.

Breastfeeding

Many older first-time mothers want to breastfeed and succeed even if it takes time to settle into an easy routine. However, some women don't want to breastfeed and others can't. Sue, for example, had to take a drug for an earlier stroke which precluded breastfeeding. If you don't breastfeed, don't feel bad about it. Babies thrive on bottled milk too and you shouldn't feel, as some women do, that you are failing your child.

Some of the best moments for appreciating the cuddliness of your new baby at first are likely to be during feeding, especially after a feed. There is something wonderful about the drowsy scrunched-up face and the warm milky smell of a satisfied baby and fathers ought to be able to share that too (try passing the baby over to your partner sometimes straight after a feed). One enormous advantage of bottle feeding, of course, is that he, or someone else, can feed her.

The time it takes It is easy enough to take in the information that demand feeding can mean six or eight feeds a day but not everybody realizes how long that can take. I had not understood that although the baby takes enough milk for nourishment in the first 5–7 minutes of sucking, my baby (and many others) might like to suck for an hour if I would let him and be pretty unhappy if I wouldn't. How you feel about that 'comfort sucking' will depend on whether you find it a close, pleasurable thing and therefore a lovely opportunity for a rest – watching television, reading or chatting. On the other hand you may wish she would stop so you can get on with the next thing. No prizes for guessing which of the two will do you most good, but it's not always easy to feel that.

Establishing the milk supply It has been suggested, and it may be suggested to you, that it takes longer for the milk supply to become established in older women – as much as six or eight weeks. This certainly happens to some women but probably has more to do with anxiety, expecting to fit too much into a day and insufficient rest, than mere age. When I tried to find out more about this, Peggy Thomas, General Secretary of the Association of Breastfeeding Mothers, wrote to me:

> I have never heard of any research to support the claim that older women take more time to establish their milk supply. I have certainly heard the claim, however, and am convinced it's a rationale put forward to explain breastfeeding failure. This is caused, in all age groups, by misinformation and lack of support. My advice to a so-called older woman would be to take good care of yourself, and don't be bamboozled by people exhorting you to get up, get dressed and get going.

If you do find that you don't have enough milk (and that often happens in the early evening, especially if you are a bit tired and low) try to spend most of the next day in bed with your baby, eating and drinking things you like, resting and enjoying being with her. Let her feed whenever she likes and suck for as long as she likes to bring your supply up to the level of her demands. It will be a lot easier to do this for a whole day if you don't try to do anything else at all and you'll probably both enjoy it.

Total breastfeeding The trend towards total breastfeeding is vigorous and the arguments are convincing – breast milk *is* best for babies and it is very convenient, at the right temperature and free from germs. Much more than that, it is a source of immense pleasure and enjoyment for you and your baby. Breastfeeding is also eminently flexible, as Lynne found.

> The first time I went out for the evening was to an NCT film evening. There was no way Matthew would have slept through the whole evening but I thought if I sat on the back row no one would notice in the dark if Matt woke up and I fed him. The inevitable happened and halfway through the film he woke up. I surreptitiously lifted my jumper but Matthew couldn't find my nipple in the dark and made slurpy lip-smacking sounds which seemed to echo even louder in the darkness. Everybody laughed. Of course they realized what was going on and I realized how silly I was to mind feeding in public and it has never bothered me since.

Not all women find that breastfeeding suits them all of the time and there's nothing wrong in admitting that. You may be going back to work soon (in which case, see p. 201) or you may find it is simply too much of a tie to spend so much time feeding. The breastfeeding movement may seem a bit purist in some respects and I certainly regret now that I refused to use a bottle at all, even when I was patently short of milk. As we have already said, the great advantage of an alternative method of feeding is that another person can feed the baby. Apart from giving you a welcome break this can be a great pleasure for a father who may feel excluded by total breastfeeding. Clem put it this way:

> When you've tried to do absolutely everything, like change him and cuddle him and walk up and down, in the last resort if he was hungry, you had a really big problem. There was this funny mild feeling of rejection. He's screaming at you and you think, What the hell are you doing this for? Give me a break. I *can't* feed you. There might have been times when I could have used a bottle. That would have been quite nice.

Mixing breast and bottle An occasional bottle doesn't harm the baby and as long as you wait a couple of weeks for her to get used to the breast, it doesn't mean she will then prefer the teat. You do need to offer the bottle quite early on:

> I wish that I'd known how easy it is to express breast milk with a little hand pump and that I had done this into a bottle. Then he could have had my milk without my being so sore and I could have had a good night's sleep. I should have given him breast milk from a bottle earlier because he hated it when I tried one at three months and I was desperate as I was going back to work.

Some women find it off-puttingly slow to use a breast pump. You might find it easier to use a Kanesan pump (which is like an inverted bottle with a vacuum) available from chemists or from the NCT breastfeeding counsellor.

If you want to continue breastfeeding but would like to use a bottle as well on a regular basis, it is better to express your own milk for the first couple of months until your supply is well established. Using formula milk to satisfy the baby's hunger if you don't have enough milk should be done in exceptional circumstances only in the first weeks – as a last resort if you feel at the end of your tether. Preferably you should offer that bottle after a normal breastfeed so that the sucking will still stimulate your supply.

Trusting your judgement Getting the feeding right for your own baby will come with practical experience and the more confident about trusting your judgement you can be, the easier it is. Maureen felt confused:

> With my first baby, since I knew nothing, I assumed everyone else must know better, e.g. health visitor, doctor, relatives, etc. So I tried to take all their advice which was mostly conflicting and got nowhere fast. I found in the end it was much better to follow my own instincts and watch my baby and get to know him and find out what was required that way.

Marian puts that sort of point of view even more strongly:

> *Everyone* has theories on child rearing. Don't take any notice. Trust to instinct. If it feels right, do it. You'll soon find out if you were wrong and then you won't try that one again.

Jacky felt she would do much better next time:

> If I had another baby I wouldn't make such a performance out of every feed. I was very rigid about the length of time she sucked and I used to change her nappy at every feed. In the middle of the night, when she'd sucked herself back to sleep I would disturb her to change her nappy and then wonder why she took so long to settle.

Night feeds It is quite common for breastfed babies to wake for a feed during the night two or three times for as long as a year. Lynne, who has already described how Matthew slept in their bed, felt that he was much more confident if his needs were met.

> Some night feeds were very special, just us two alone in the velvety darkness, no distractions, and we might have been the only two people in the whole world awake at that time. Yet I knew that there would be other mothers awake feeding their babies all over the world and I felt a special bond with them.

There is no need for it always to be just the two of you. Angela:

> For the first two months of her life Victoria performed at night like a cabaret turn. The small hours were party time. While her arms and legs churned the air like mini helicopter

propellers, Tony and I sat beside her on the bedroom floor drinking Guinness straight from the bottle and sometimes munching sandwiches.

It is worth starting very early to introduce the idea that nights are for sleeping by putting the baby to sleep in a darkened room and keeping night-time contact as brief and low key as possible. This could save you battles once it gets to the time that you hope she might start sleeping through.

Crying

Your baby will let you know when she's hungry by crying but she will probably also cry for other reasons and it isn't always easy to know why. One study suggests that all first babies cry more and sleep less than their mothers expected.[2] Some mothers cry more than they expected too! There is also an idea that older mothers find it harder to cope with their baby's crying than some younger mothers. This may have something to do with their longer experience of rational behaviour – they try to account for the crying more precisely and feel anxious when they can't. But even if you do know why your baby is crying, you can't always do anything about it and that can be hard to bear. Jacky:

> I was used to being in a situation over which I almost always had control. Now, suddenly, there was this tiny mite whose slightest squeal would set me sweating and feeling panicky and sick. Nobody could help me because nobody could actually come and take it all from me. I don't think I was actually depressed but I do think I was overwhelmed with the feeling that it was almost too much to cope with – not the practical things like nappies, washing, cooking, cleaning – those things I dealt with and in fact enjoyed as a sort of therapy. My main source of concern was what to do when the baby cried in between feeds.

Lack of feedback The lack of feedback at the beginning is difficult. As you get to know your baby, you start to recognize what her crying means, even if you can't always stop her. You learn that she is hungry or uncomfortable, in pain or lonely. In the first weeks you haven't got that far yet and you don't *know* you're doing all right. Your baby can't say, 'Look, I'm really OK even if

I do cry all the time.' For older women, who have become used to being able to measure how well they are doing in a variety of ways, this is a difficult adjustment. In many jobs if something matters and you work hard enough you can achieve your aim. It isn't like that with babies – you can spend all your time and energy feeding, changing, rocking, singing to your baby and sometimes she will *still* yell.

As you get used to it, you find ways of dealing with what the crying means. Janice:

> The twins hated being bathed though I found out that if you wrap a nervous or newborn baby in a clean nappy and then lower the whole thing into the bath, they don't get frightened.

Sue wasn't expecting the strong biological pull of her baby's crying:

> I thought, I shall be strict, I shall let him cry. But I don't seem to be able to do that. Three minutes and I've had it. It makes me really uptight and emotional and I just want to pick him up.

Evening crying Many babies have a restless time in the evening when they cry a lot and seem unable to settle. For some, but not all, it may be colic. It is absolutely the worst time for you – you are tired and looking forward to the time of day that used to be yours, after work, when you could relax, eat, chat to your partner. It sometimes feels as if she's doing it on purpose to get at you when you're down. If it does get you down, ask a friend to look after her for an hour or two and go out for a drink or go off on your own somewhere out of earshot. Your friends probably won't mind your baby's crying nearly as much as you do and not only because they know they can give her back.

Crying in the night Unquestionably, the worst kind of crying is that which goes on in the middle of the night when the only thing you want to do is go to sleep yourself. Marian, who had to cope with Daniel on her own, offers these methods for getting your fretful baby to sleep:

1 Wrap tightly in a shawl.
2 Cradle in arms and rock to sleep.

3 Sing lullaby – any old words will do – the more interesting the better for *your* sake. The baby only needs your voice and rhythmic tones.

4 Lay the baby on her tummy – bang her bum firmly and steadily – they say one thump per second. Lay the other hand on her shoulder then gradually decrease pressure.

5 Lay her on her tummy – rub back firmly and rhythmically.

6 Put babe over shoulder, wrapped in shawl – bang bum or pat to sleep.

7 Overcome strong crying by very fierce rocking – very exaggerated movements.

8 Some people recommend turning on the hoover.

9 Put babe in pram and rock to sleep.

10 Give up: get up, make coffee, pretend it's day and assume she will not return to sleep this night!

The rewards

It may seem obvious to say that the kind of baby you will have will affect the sort of start you have. If your baby has colic, she will cry. If she is restless and gets bored easily or has difficulty getting to sleep, she will be more demanding. And, despite what one might like to believe, boys do seem to be more active and demanding than a lot of girls. Babies vary tremendously in the amount of sleep they need – one study revealed that 'at birth the time spent asleep per day ranged from eight to 16 hours'.[3]

If you get a contented baby you are very lucky. The first weeks were made much easier for Alice, a single mother:

> The good thing was that she wasn't a cry-cry baby. I could feed her when it's time to feed her, dress her, change her and put her down and she'd be very happy.

Sally also had a lovely start:

> It was a very very happy time for me. It never occurred to me not to be completely absorbed and fulfilled by every minor detail. I didn't need anything else except seeing people. It was a bit strange really and I'm not sure how but I felt very confident and in control of what I was doing and that it was working. It's a bit *not* how it's supposed to be. Thomas was a very easy baby.

But even if your baby isn't particularly easy, looking after her can be a very positive experience. Janice felt like this after her twins were born:

> I wish I'd known how *rewarding* such strange little objects as newborn babies can be. They couldn't focus their eyes, they looked like skinned rabbits and yet the twins enthralled us. I'm sure that the so-called 'wind smile' is really to give the parents pleasure until such time as the baby can smile deliberately!

It is easy to dwell on the difficult things and, indeed, problems need to be talked over and ways found of dealing with them. No one has much difficulty dealing with happiness, but the thing about feeling good is that it can be so intimate and personal that any expression of it can sound like a cliché. Sue found the first weeks hard but said: 'I don't think you could ever go through such a catastrophic thing if it wasn't so wonderful. I think the whole thing is so amazing.'

These are the words that people use all the time – amazing, wonderful, marvellous, fantastic. But the words can't carry the meaning. They are not just expressions of joy. You may *truly* find your baby amazing in that she really does amaze you; you may feel genuinely full of wonderment and marvel at her. It is a new and complete feeling for you and terribly hard to share with anyone else without going over the top. But it rides beneath all the difficulties as the strength and the core that makes all those other things not just tolerable, but surmountable, because there's a reason for them and what you've got in the end is your lovely baby. The intensity of feeling is hard to share but so is the feeling that it is very private. Paul:

> You're anxious that you could become a bore, because everyone else has gone through the same process, whether it was 14 years ago or two. So what to you is unique and exciting and phenomenal is fairly commonplace. That comes over fairly soon. So then you share your joy and amazement with each other but not with other people because they'd gone through it themselves.

Rebecca, a single mother, said that one of the hardest things for her about bringing her twins up on her own was *not* being able to share the little details that increase the enjoyment so much.

The intimacy Because of the way men's work is arranged, the mother spends much more time with her baby than most fathers do, though work isn't the only reason for that. You have the pleasure of getting to know her really well – the smiles for you, the chuckles as you learn where she really likes being tickled, the day when instead of screaming every time she has her nappy changed, she lies staring at you quietly, seeming not to blink. The gradual recognition of her special smell, particularly when she's sleeping. Looking at your baby sleeping peacefully must be one of the most moving experiences in the world – her vulnerability, hands limply flopped above her head. You also get to know her so well because you do so much for her. Aleid likes that: 'What I like about it is that it is so basic. There's no theorizing. There's no shall I or shan't I? All the things simply need doing. I really enjoy that – it's so down to earth. It's all those basic things about food, about cleaning, basic human things that need doing and you do them.' It is often the small, intimate details that last as part of the most positive memories. Maggie:

There were very few problems in the first few weeks. I was surprised at how quickly I was fit again. The most positive things about being new parents were:

1 Being filled with wonder at the perfectness of the tiny human being we had managed to create between us.
2 A new sense of responsibility and increased awareness of our importance to each other.
3 Lovely sunny days, picnics on the lawn, nappies and tiny washing hanging on the line.
4 The overwhelming number of gifts and cards – such kindness from people including ones we hardly thought we knew.
5 'Picnics' during the night – feedtimes we made enjoyable with Horlicks and biscuits.
6 Philip's reluctance to go to work – he wanted to stay at home with us (finally persuaded him we needed the money!).
7 Walking into the village pub for the first time after the birth to receive a standing ovation from the locals.

In the same way that Philip was reluctant to go back to work,

other men were surprised by the intensity of pleasure they got
from their baby. Robert:

> We were both relaxed in handling and cuddling and because
> Chris was happy to let me do most of the cuddling, I spent a
> lot of time physically handling, hugging and cuddling. We are
> still extremely close, physically, today. (Henry is now two.) I
> remember the first few weeks as ones of suppressing natural
> anxieties. Every cough, sneeze, cry had to be explained,
> rationalized. I checked for cot death several times a night –
> gradually forcing myself to show less concern and indeed be
> less concerned. I enjoyed changing him from the beginning. I
> loved holding him, feeling his grip. My overall memory is one
> of great happiness, joy, pride and of overwhelming love.

Your rights

To remind yourself of benefits and rights now that the baby is
born, see p. 65.

7

How You Feel about Yourself

However the birth affects you, you are bound to feel different. It might be lovely, the difference, or it might be quite bewildering and hard to cope with. Because you are over 30 you've had years of living without a baby and there are all sorts of changes and adjustments to be made. Sue:

> For 15 years of my life I hadn't had to think of anybody but me. I wasn't prepared for the immense shock of having a baby – this 'thing' that I had to look after all the time. I'd had a very selfish life up to that point. I found it very hard that you can't just go away, break away, without making loads of arrangements. Having him outweighs all of that but sometimes I do wish that I was just on my own again.

Aleid:

> I'd be walking in the street and I'd think 'Gosh – I've got a baby. I'm a mother.' I still feel that sometimes. I'm walking in the street and I think, 'Look it's *me*.' My life has changed dramatically in the last three years and I love it.

Heather:

> I feel there is a real me – the person who goes to work and reads the books I want to read and watches the TV programmes I want to watch and does all the things I want to

do – which is in constant conflict with this other person who is having to do mostly domestic chores. I don't see motherhood in negative terms. What it comes down to is that the person who is me is being swallowed up by the person who is mother.

How quickly and how readily you adapt to being a mother is bound to depend on how you feel about yourself once you become one. Holding on to a sense of 'me' sometimes needs a conscious effort. This chapter will look at some of the adjustments that need to be made when you become a first-time mother over 30. They won't all apply to you but they are based on the varied experiences of women who have all had their first babies after 30. Asking questions of yourself might help you to home in on those experiences that tie in with your own or examine and think about issues you may as yet be only vaguely aware of.

Do you have an image of what a 'good mother' should be?

Your experience of life by now will probably have made you sceptical enough of the cosy media images of smiling, competent mothers with adorable babies and of the propaganda (growing apace with unemployment) that babies need their mothers to look after them all the time. That is out there and can be dismissed at an intellectual level at least. But when you are groping about for reassurance, you may turn to what you think will help. Vicky:

> None of the booklets provided by the hospital or the health visitor mentioned babies who did not sleep. *All* the babies had good sleeping habits and they all had good feeding routines. The mothers in the books were the same fairy tale ladies as the ones in TV commercials. I wish I hadn't expected so much of myself and expected to carry on as before I had my baby.

You might well have an image of what a good mother is that rejects the established cosiness but that makes heavy demands on you all the same. Women over 30 often take their role as mothers extremely seriously, possibly more seriously than a younger woman. If you have become used to analysing your actions, thinking ahead, weighing up the pros and cons, evaluating your own performance, you may trust less to instinct and gut-reaction than someone with less experience would have to do. That can be double-edged: you may get more out of it all but you might also be less easily satisfied and harder on yourself than is either appropriate or good for you. Anna said, 'I think I tried too hard to be a perfect mother, which led to guilt feelings when I had to keep him waiting or felt irritated with him.' Looking back Kay also felt she had tried too hard:

> I tended to get a bit over-anxious and try and do the right thing. I'm aware of just how responsible I am, how important being a parent is and bringing up a healthy well-adjusted being. I've seen so many in social work who aren't well-adjusted. But I've let go a lot of that now. I realize you have to be natural and give what you can. But to begin with I thought I must keep him stimulated, not let him cry too long and all this carry-on. Now I think, God, if I'd had three I'd never have time to worry. You just have to get on with it.

One of the trends in advice on child-rearing is to get mothers to see things from the baby's point of view – Penelope Leach, for example, is superbly good at this and offers a helpful perspective.[1] But it does encourage you not to think about yourself much and to set yourself very high sights as to what a 'good mother' should do and feel. I found it helpful to remind myself of a concept developed by Donald Winnicott, the child psychologist – that of 'good-enough mothering'. It takes in the idea that you accept your responsibilities and that you want to love and care for your child well but to be a 'good-enough' mother allows some room for manoeuvre and, more important, some leeway for *you*. In other words, helpless and demanding though she may be, your baby doesn't *always* have to come first. Sometimes you must do what you want to do even if it means interrupting her routine or making her wait. She has to fit in with your life too – the danger of the 'good mother' syndrome is that the baby *becomes* your life.

How do you define yourself?

How you feel about yourself is bound to be influenced by whether you have decided to return to your job or to become a full-time mother. Both of these situations will be dealt with in some detail in chapters 10 and 11. If you have given up your job (even temporarily) and have no fixed plans for the future other than looking after your baby, you might, like Gill, feel anxious about how that will work:

> It worried me that I wouldn't be happy staying at home. I didn't know how I would react to the lack of independence, the lack of status. I enjoyed the responsibility of the work I did and I enjoyed functioning as me quite independently of Tim or anyone else. Suddenly I realized that I wouldn't be able to do that again for a long time because I would always be someone's mother, then someone's wife, then me.

To some extent Gill's sense of her self had been defined through her work. If someone said 'What do you do?' she said she was a teacher. For women who have been working for 10 or 15 years, especially in one specific sphere, it can be a strange feeling not to have that clear sense of who you are now. Anna:

> One of the biggest adjustments is finding a new identity, not only one to present to the outside world but also internally. I'm still not quite sure who I am now. Certainly I don't feel inside myself that my place in life is defined in terms of being Neil's mum, though I think I do accept the realities of my situation – which is that at present every day is virtually devoted to looking after Neil and keeping the house going. I try to keep a finger on my outside 'work' but at present it's pretty much a token, though all the more important for that. So I read the newspaper each day plus at least one specialist magazine and find that I have almost no time left for 'fun reading' and I do miss just being able to sink into a book.

Do other people treat you differently?

Many women mentioned with pleasure that they felt they had joined a sort of club when they had a baby. Helena felt very proud of Josh: 'I like going out to places with him. When you go into shops and up to the cash desk, it's completely different from when you used to go shopping on your own. People say hello and want to talk to him and talk to you and ask how old he is. It's quite different.' Strangers talk to you at bus stops and in shops and some other strangers stop talking to you. Annie:

> I quite enjoy the anonymity that having a baby gives you.

When you're a single woman you get a lot of hassle – stupid things like men whistling at you in the street. You do feel quite conscious of being a woman on your own. I find it very nice to have a buggy and walk around. You just don't get it any more. I didn't expect that to happen.

The friendly even admiring acceptance of you as a mother gives a warm comfortable feeling but it is very generalized. You also need social contact on your pre-mother level and if that changes it can be a surprise. Sue:

When I was pregnant we went out an awful lot and then it was more and more difficult to go out. Loads of people came round but I noticed a great change in my life. I *used* to have an intellectual conversation with them but all of a sudden we had a different relationship. I wanted to say let's talk about something other than this child.

If you are going to preserve the self that was you before you had your baby you need to build in some time to do other things quite deliberately and quite early on. Marge:

I first went out for two hours in the evening when the baby was three weeks old. My husband baby-sat and it was good for both of us. By leaving him on his own with the baby he can't be worried that I'm watching him or be anxious as to how he's handling Joe. Having a baby at my age I think I am more able to cope and have confidence to do things as and when I feel it's right. If I had been younger I might not have had the confidence to try and retain my social life.

Have you hung on to your confidence?

Lots of women said that they lost confidence in themselves after having their baby and this is very common amongst all mothers. Older women might feel it more strongly, though, having had so much more time to build up confidence in the first place. Those women whose confidence arose from the work they did felt it most if they ended up looking after their babies in an isolated and lonely environment. Being with other people for at least some of the time helps enormously but it needs to be a real relationship, not just the superficial contact you get from friendly shoppers. Alice could have had a very lonely start as a mother – she is a single parent, was unemployed for a year after her baby was born and had very little money. But she belonged to a black women's group:

> When the group came about I was one of the founder members. I'd just had my baby then and it was very important for me. There are things like supplementary education, a craft shop of mainly African and West Indian crafts, a tuck shop and they do hair plaiting – hence the hair style! It's open from about 10.30. There's a dance group and we fight campaigns – I'm on the campaign committee. So it's a mixture of all sorts. I think having a baby has made me more responsible. But I don't think I've changed my opinion of myself. If anything I've become more confident in myself. Whereas before, if anyone was ill or an accident happened, I'd just panic and run. Now I'm faced with a situation where I've got to stand and face it and that has helped me to have confidence in myself.

Isolated in her council flat with a small baby and no money, Alice's life could have been very different.

How much support do you get?

Having the support of other women who know what it's like is enormously helpful. On one level the practical talk about how babies develop and the hints you pick up from each other is reassuring and useful. On another, knowing that other people share the doubts or conflicts or difficulties in adjusting helps too. But it isn't easy to find the right people to share these thoughts – the women's groups that do function for mothers, the National Childbirth Trust coffee mornings, the National Housewives Register meetings, can't by their very nature offer that closeness or intimacy. There needs to be a chance to talk on that second level but you might have to create the chance yourself through friends you already have or new ones you make. Margaret:

> I think it's very difficult to have a coherent image of oneself both as feminist and mother (and wife). I know lots of feminists are mothers but the single, or even lesbian ones, get the limelight. This area remains largely unexplored by the women's movement would-be theorists – if not positively disdained, but it seems to me to be of great importance. I feel

all my spare energy at present is going into resolving the conflicts personally and in a way that is a waste of energy.

The area Margaret describes is changing and perhaps becoming less exclusively personal. Many of the women who are having their babies after 30 are feminists and encourage each other: Helena:

> A lot of the women that I know who are friends are also feminists and have children. I suppose I've been able to go ahead and have a child because I've felt that it was all right – I knew that other women had managed to do it and still retained their feminist views. I can't think of anyone I know who was a feminist who has changed her outlook as a result of having a baby. When I was 29 I had an abortion – I didn't know many other women here and I wasn't courageous enough to go ahead with it. Later, having the house helped and I was influenced by a friend who had a baby – I thought if she can, so can I.

Like Alice, Helena feels that she is now more confident than she was before. They both clearly got some of their strength from other women.

Making the Adjustments

Retaining your sense of identity, your confidence and having the opportunity to share your new feelings and experiences with other people who know what it's like, all help you to feel good (or better) about yourself. The time at which you feel like reasserting your own identity may differ from woman to woman. Katherine:

> I felt quite clear about what I expected (and thought I was expected) to do for about seven months. All this time I was breastfeeding and felt that the baby and I were a complete unit. When I started to wean him it was partly because I wanted to have my own body back again after all that time of pregnancy and breastfeeding. But when I had weaned him I realized he was 'completely' separate and I had to rediscover/ redefine who I was, and it was quite a difficult period of transition.

For other women, this may come a lot earlier, or later when the child starts to go to playgroup or nursery school.

Using your expertise

During your adult life and particularly in your working life you will have developed ways of looking at the world and ways of getting things done. These can work against you as well as for you but the more aware you are of *how* they work, the more positive use you can make of them. Marian:

> I am extremely methodical and obsessive about detail. It is exactly the same with Daniel but I consciously build in easy-goingness. I try to be as flexible as possible over the pattern of his day and how he wants to feed, sleep, etc. I try to follow his pace and suggest patterns to him, rather than impose them. I've tried to provide the very detailed framework of his life.

Moira:

> In both philosophy and linguistics it helps if you can approach your data from as many angles as possible and within as open mind as possible: when I remember, I find it also helps with looking after my child.

Flexibility is vitally important and it might not be one of your strengths. Lesley:

> As a teacher I was good at administration and organization and when there are tons of jobs to be done at home I enjoy the sense of being a manager and planning my day. But the disadvantage of this is that I find it *very* frustrating when I don't achieve what I want to achieve, when jobs are only half done and not done properly. Being a perfectionist is a serious disadvantage with a baby. I have had to learn to be flexible and not to plan too much. I had been used to a strictly timetabled existence, meeting deadlines, making lists and getting the jobs done. Now I have a tiny dependent creature who prevents me finishing almost any job when I want to.

Monica found that her training as a probation officer helped her:

I have found some of the concepts used to analyse personal relationships and situations useful. For example, I felt very resentful towards my baby in the first days and it occurred to me that I had moved overnight from a highly dependent and helpless situation to having a baby dependent and helpless on me. Therefore, a kind of emotional jet lag seemed inevitable. I was aware of having very short-term goals in order not to get frustrated, e.g. today I will mop the floor/do the washing/make a cake and as long as I did, I was satisfied.

Maintaining your social life

Your social life is bound to change quite dramatically but here it does seem to help to be older. Several people mentioned missing the spontaneity of going out for a last minute drink or to see a film but by and large there is very little feeling that you might be missing out on something. You are more likely to have old friends of long standing if you are over 30 and seeing these people is likely to mean more to you than anything else. It is worth trying quite hard to see that you don't cut yourself off from them even if it may not be easy to keep in touch. While the baby is very small it is quite possible to take her with you to other people's houses, restaurants, meetings. As she gets more settled into her own routine at about six months and recognizes her own home as being special, it can become more difficult. It may be worth training your child to sleep in other places, especially if you are a single parent, but it doesn't always work. Some children just don't do that happily.

Being aware of your needs

Jane well describes the dilemmas of many mothers:

What I remember most of all was the grim determination to make some part of every day my own, so that I could do my own thing. Looking back it was almost impossible; trying to force my brain to click into action as two wailing children walked off with a 19-year-old girl I hired for two hours every afternoon – knowing that I had deadlines to meet and that the two hours was all I would get till the next day – and at the same time feeling awful guilt and longing to throw down my pen and run after them and behave like a normal mother.

Of course, a 'normal' mother wouldn't have wanted to do something for herself at all, she'd have wanted to take the children to the park herself every afternoon. Those attitudes, romantic and nostalgic as they are, dig deep.

Getting some time for yourself

One of the things that older women miss most after having a baby is having some time *alone* just being by yourself. Unless you are very unusual, you will need time on your own without your child and that doesn't happen by itself. You need to be able to look forward to it and count on it. So you need to set it up. What you choose to do with that time doesn't matter and will depend on what is important to you. You may just want to potter about; you may go to work or work at home; you may read a book or go shopping; you may go swimming or have a long bath. You do need to be able to renew yourself. Looking after babies and small children is extremely rewarding but it is hard work and if you don't get a break it becomes less rewarding. No one would expect you to do a full-time job of any other kind without a coffee or lunch break or the occasional day off.

The earlier you can get used to *leaving the baby with someone else* the easier it is for both of you. At first, if you're breastfeeding, you won't be able to do it for very long, but even an hour or two makes a difference. Your baby needs to get used to the fact that if you leave her you will come back. You will be a very special person to her from the start but if you spend most of your day with her, every day, you become more and more special. By the time she is six or seven months old you are so special that she can hardly bear it if you do leave her unless she is already used to it. If you are working you'll have to make some arrangements anyway. The options open to you are dealt with in chapter 11.

Encourage your partner to spend time with the baby. Build in regular slots when you both know this will happen. She's his baby too, and even if he comes in tired from work, you're tired too. At weekends especially you should also have some free time. Quite apart from the good it does you, he needs to spend time with her if he is going to be an effective father and it will be better for all of you if some of that time is spent on their own together.

You might have *a relative or friend or neighbour* whom you could ask or who might offer to look after the baby for a couple of hours. Try to let the baby get used to the same people because then, as she grows up, they will be part of the familiar circle of people she can trust when you're not there. It is very good for her to have contact with adults other than her parents and it's good for the adults too. In other words, you could be doing them a favour not the other way around.

If you go to events or places that have a crèche and you would like to use one, start early – at least by three or four months, so that it isn't new and bewildering for the baby later on.

There might be a *babysitting circle* in your neighbourhood and if there isn't, you might start one. Usually these operate with a group of parents who babysit for each other and exchange tokens instead of money. Find out about daytime babysitting. Some people might be happy to look after your baby during the day and you can then pay them back by sitting at night. Going out to babysit can be a real luxury if your partner looks after your baby for you – it is your time to read or write letters or watch television or do any of the things there's never time for at home.

There might be *teenagers* in your neighbourhood who are prepared to look after the baby for a small amount of money. At first you might like to stay at home, doing something in another room, until you feel they've got to know your baby. I had a set-up like that which proved a real saving grace as Ben grew older. By the time he was two, the two teenage sisters who lived round the corner thought of him as their little brother and came to see him most days after school, which was lovely for me.

Arranging a *swap* with a friend is a very useful way of getting some time off. More details of how to make a system like this work are given in chapter 10.

Getting your sleep

You renew yourself by your own activities but also by sleeping. How much sleep you get usually depends on luck – on how much and how well your baby sleeps. Pauline:

> On the whole our way of life physically hasn't changed as much as we'd expected. Everyone who knew us muttered dire warnings about 'Oh you won't have any more mornings in bed at weekends.' But Rosie has proved the most adaptable baby – at weekends she often doesn't get her breakfast until 11 or 12 and will be happily playing in her cot until then.

Lucky Pauline. I still remember reading that with incredible
envy because it came at a time when Ben was waking three, four
or five times every night and once and for all at 5.30 every
morning. Kay found that lack of sleep reduced her enjoyment: 'I
got a bit frightened because I found my reasoning wasn't as good
as it should have been. I wasn't thinking straight. I would forget
things. I'd be in a conversation with somebody and I would
suddenly go off and they'd say "Hey!" I think it's lack of sleep
more than anything that does that.'

If at three or four months your baby is still waking you on a
regular basis or if she has a period of sleeping through the night
and then regresses, it is worth trying to do something about it. It
might mean committing yourself to a plan of action that feels
slightly out of kilter with your style with the baby but if that
means you get fewer disturbed nights it will be worth it. In their
book *My Child Won't Sleep* Jo Douglas and Naomi Richman
suggest ways of dealing with sleep problems.[2] Their advice seems
eminently sane and useful. Based on a self-help analysis of
sleeping patterns and a suggested management programme, I
wish it had been available when Ben was little.

How you feel about your baby

You will almost certainly feel charmed and enchanted by your
baby, deeply moved by her helplessness and fragile beauty and
increasingly fascinated by the changes as she develops and
grows. But you probably won't feel like that all the time and the
pleasure you get out of her will be affected by the sort of baby she
is and how you feel about small babies. A number of women said
that their partners started relating much better to their babies as
they got older – they didn't get so much out of a small baby who
couldn't respond much. Some *women* feel that too but it isn't so
acceptable to admit it. Since several women said that one of the
reasons they had delayed having a child until they were over 30
was because they weren't 'particularly baby minded', this may
be even more true of older women. If you are the person held
responsible for looking after the baby, it's too bad if you really
prefer toddlers or older children. Luckily they grow up very fast!

The baby you get is a matter of chance to some extent,
although of course she will pick up vibrations from you. Some
babies sleep a lot, others don't. Some get colic, others don't.
Some cry a lot, others coo and gurgle happily. What your baby is

like will make a big difference to you and there's no question that if she sleeps well and is contented and peaceful when awake, she'll be much easier to look after.

If you are unlucky and get a difficult, demanding baby it can be hard to cope. The temptation is to blame yourself and say, 'If I was different, so would she be.' That almost certainly isn't true and doesn't help at all. Even if your baby is picking up some tension from you (as we are so often told) there may not be much you can do about it and it becomes a vicious circle. What would probably help most is to get away from her for a while to break the pattern. Katherine:

> A thought about those moments when you feel you can't cope with your baby, when there seems no reason for her being upset and cross and you've tried all the food, sleep, changing possibilities: I remember developing two contrasting tactics. One was to put him in his cot and let us both have a few moments away from each other – and quite often he calmed down – but even if he didn't, I did! The other was the opposite – to give him more direct attention – playing with him rather than hoping he would entertain himself while I was getting on with other things and only giving him half my attention. These responses probably related to quite different moods of his, and the latter became more common as he got older. But it seemed to make sense (a) that he should sometimes get fed up with me, (b) that sometimes I should just admit I couldn't cope and remove myself, and (c) that half an hour or an hour's direct play and then bed or food or whatever was much more satisfying for us both than two hours of half-attention and a lot of grizzling.

Resentment You will not be unusual if you sometimes feel irritated and resentful. Jacky:

> One of the hardest adjustments to make was that of coming to terms with the fact that my life and my time were no longer my own. I could resent it if she woke up while I was trying to read, write, watch TV, etc. I felt she was impinging on my privacy. Of course all this made me feel guilty too, that I should resent her at all. I think that perhaps is the major factor in having a first child over 30 – adjusting takes longer. Now, after two years of motherhood, I think I've just about sorted it out and no longer feel that my time is being wasted if I've spent an afternoon playing with Alice.

I remember vividly the first time I ever felt really resentful of Ben. It was about three weeks after the birth and I still wasn't well. Clem was at home and after lunch we both went to bed, in separate rooms so as not to disturb each other. I was dreadfully tired and had looked forward to this rest all morning. Just as I snuggled down, I heard Ben cry. Instead of calling Clem, which is what I should have done, I got up. It was fairly clear that Ben was going to stay awake so I took him downstairs and we sat in front of the fire.

It was an important time for me. The only thing I wanted was to sleep. I felt extremely resentful – of Ben for waking just at that moment, of Clem for sleeping when I couldn't. I looked at the tiny, alert, grumpy baby, lost in the middle of his brown bouncing chair and was overcome by that sense of his dependence and my responsibility that everyone talks about. I felt it as a physical dragging, sinking sensation, deep down. This creature would be dependent on me for a very long time, would continue to stop me doing what I wanted at times; at other times would stop me doing what I needed to do, like sleep. And I had to get used to all that. Of course I can see now that I should have expected Clem to get used to it too!

Feeling responsible No matter how much responsibility you are used to, and by the time you are over 30 that might be considerable, there is nothing quite like the feeling of responsibility that comes with a baby. It can be quite overwhelming. Judy:

> I loved my son from the moment I saw him but even that welling up of emotion did not give me the self-confidence to deal with the task I had taken on. In fact, I think that because I loved him so tenderly I was all the more horrified by my responsibility. I really felt that he could not survive without me personally and that I was not up to the task. Had I been younger I don't think I would have agonized so. There is a very necessary arrogancce in youth that helps deal with many things.

Even when every effort is made to share the responsibility, it does seem to be different for women. Cathy and John tried to share looking after Claire in an organized way by each working part-time but Cathy still doesn't find it easy: 'It's much easier for

John to walk out of the front door than me. That dependence I find very hard work. I think one of the reasons I don't have any mental energy for anything else in adjusting to having somebody so dependent on me. It seems to fill my whole head.' This is clearly a shared feeling. Fiona: 'There is a slight feeling of tension all the time, a knowledge that one can never completely relax. One always has this tremendous responsibility, one must never be late, never be ill, never drink too much. I think this is the greatest adjustment of all.'

Knowing yourself and working things out

As your child gets older and can understand and respond to your feelings as well as demanding that you attend to hers, the fact that you know yourself and how you operate can help you in your dealings with her. Because you are over 30 you're probably fairly self-aware and can use your understanding positively. Alice has certainly found this in spite of the difficulties of bringing her daughter up on her own:

> I've enjoyed it so far. I think if you're aware of your temperament a lot of trouble can be avoided. If I'm tired and in a bad mood because I'm tired I won't just sit there and knock her to pieces. We're at the stage when we understand each other (she's four and a half now) so I'd say, 'Look, I'm tired and really I could do with a sleep. So if you don't mind, when you're ready, you tell me the same thing.' I think I enjoy it because I've got so much out of it. I've become more responsible, I've become more calm and it's only through having a child. I've become much more aware of children's needs and because I'm *learning* from it, it's helping me to help her.

How you feel about the future

The responsibility of being the central generation creates its own worries and questions, especially about the future. Several older parents say that they feel quite differently about the world now that they have a child. Jacky:

> I try not to think about the future at all – it terrifies me. Only since becoming a mother have I really begun to fear the future

at all. Somehow before Alice, I could accept the possibilities of nuclear war, economic slump or whatever with a somewhat philosophical fear. But now I've joined the peace movement and will do anything to prevent a holocaust.

Looking on the most positive side, perhaps the children of the many parents who feel like Jacky, will grow up more aware of the issues at stake and may themselves, given a chance, be able to work for change.

There is a serious underlying anxiety amongst older parents (probably all parents) about the public and political future. Concern is expressed about the sort of education their children will receive and what opportunities will be open to them afterwards. But almost everybody expressed very optimistic and positive feelings about their personal future with their children. They do speculate about what it will be like as they grow older, how their children will feel about them as parents when they are teenagers, how much football and camping they will be able to cope with, but those aren't serious worries. Their children clearly give them something very special to look forward to and in the recognition of how quickly time passes is also the awareness of how much there is to enjoy.

8

You and Your Partner

Nothing like all the women who have their first babies over 30 are married to the baby's father or even live with him. Some live alone, some with another woman or group of women, others in communal households. But if you live with your partner, whether man or woman, you may find that the birth of your child changes the relationship. Clem and I tried to prepare for the change by talking it over before Ben was born, acknowledging that we wouldn't be as free to do as we liked, that we would have less money because I was giving up work. But I don't think we prepared ourselves at all for the strain of simply having a third person around all the time – one who was extremely vociferous and demanding, no respecter of our need for privacy, quiet or sleep. Nor, perhaps, did we quite appreciate the intensity of feeling we would share in delighting in our baby.

The length of the relationship

Clem and I had been living together for two and a half years when Ben was born. So in some respects our relationship was relatively new. We didn't have the stabilizing background of years of shared experience and, more importantly, knowledge of each other. However, because of our previous experience we felt very positive about our future together. Second marriages and late marriages account for quite a high proportion of first births to women over 30 and those couples usually have their babies relatively quickly.

A relationship that comes late may be stronger because you know that this time it feels right. A number of people confess to wondering 'with something like panic' one man said, whether they would ever find the kind of partner with whom they could confidently have a child, knowing how that would test them both. If you form that kind of relationship in your thirties and you want a child, you may feel there's no time to waste. Paul and Sue didn't start living together until they were married and she was already pregnant then:

We're really glad we've done it. It was a positive decision, it wasn't an accident. We were both aware that we were getting older. But I do see that that's why we argue sometimes. We didn't have that time to build on and we did too many things at once – doing the house up, having a baby, living together for the first time. Getting used to all those things was difficult without another person to cope with.

However, when we do fight or argue, we can see the humorous side of it, whereas if we were 21 we'd probably split up because we might not weather the storm. We both know that there's nothing ideal out there that's going to come floating through the door. You *know* that what you've got is really good and you've just got to overcome those bad times. At least we hadn't got sick of having long, quiet evenings on our own. We hadn't had time to do that.

Some new relationships aren't quite so interdependent. Annie became pregnant by accident when she and Don had been going out together for six months. Because she had had four miscarriages in an earlier relationship, she was very keen to have the baby even though she and Don had not planned to get so seriously involved. She shares a house with three other women:

Don was quite distressed initially because he's quite a bit younger than me, but his predominant feeling after the initial shock was that he did want to be involved. He is round here quite a lot but I don't think it would be right to force the situation where we live together because of the baby. It might do later on. I had lived with someone for three and a half years and although that was quite traumatic when it ended, I felt quite liberated by being on my own again. I see now I had been quite restricted by living with someone else. I was just beginning to feel the pleasures of living on my own. Don's friends are quite different from mine so we felt we wanted to be quite separate. We spend a lot of time together but mentally we know that we've got our own space. We work things on a day to day basis. There was a time when she was waking up a lot at night and I thought I was going loopy so he'd have her upstairs and I'd sleep downstairs.

Annie's account of why she and Don don't live together highlights some of the real difficulties faced by people who do. It isn't always easy to live with someone else especially if you have both been used to a good deal of time on your own.

Other contributors had been together for as much as ten or twelve years before having a child. That must make a difference in terms of what you've lived through together and how you cope with new or difficult times. Tim:

Gill and I certainly sorted out our relationship in the ten years before we had Rebecca. There might be an advantage in that we know one another very well and know how each will react in certain situations. We can detect when things are becoming intolerable early on without it becoming a crisis. That could be weighed against the fact that our life-style's become fairly rigid, very much a pattern to a given form, so Rebecca isn't just a variation on that pattern but an intrusion into it.

Judy and Alan had also been married for ten years when they had Justin and at first they found their own relationship very stretched. Judy:

I found that my patience was definitely finite. His incessant crying in the early months stirred emotions in me that I found very difficult to come to terms with and which aroused incredible feelings of guilt. It's very hard to admit even to oneself how bad a parent you could be. This makes it all sound very traumatic and a bit of a crisis and I suppose it was really. Alan and my relationship reached its lowest ebb. We were not used to having to share ourselves but I suppose because of the length of the relationship and how good it had been, we clung on to each other.

Sharing yourselves may well be one of the most difficult things to be faced by any couple, perhaps especially those who have had a lengthy, settled relationship. You may find the baby intrudes into some of the most precious times – enjoying a meal together at the end of the day, having a cosy lie-in on a Sunday morning, making love together. Luckily, sharing the baby herself and your mutual pleasure in the tiny changes that happen with her almost every day is compensation.

Fathers

In his book *Fatherhood*, before he started interviewing men who were about to become first-time fathers, Brian Jackson says he read everything there was available in the literature about fathers. It took about 36 working hours. To read all the relevant published material on mothers, he says, would have required 'a packed decade'. He goes on, 'The imbalance is outstanding and an index of our knowledge.'[1] So we know very little about how fathers feel. But feel they do. Paul told me:

> The first period after the initial relief of finding that he had two arms and two legs was of anxiety and wondering how well we were doing, how well *I* was doing and feeling very inadequate. It was something we had never done before and we didn't know how to do it. I knew that Sue was carrying the can for it and all I was doing was hovering somewhere in the background being relatively ineffectual.
>   Purely the right way of holding the kid became paramount. I was thinking: am I holding his head correctly, am I putting my arms in the right posture? You looked at other people who had two or three kids and they were tremendously relaxed. I over-compensated by thinking about everything. That added to the tiredness. I always remember just holding him in the first weeks. After about ten minutes I used to get pains all down my back and neck muscles. Not because he was heavy but because I was so tense trying to do the right thing.

Clem was much less tense than I was. Used to handling small animals he had no problems dressing, bathing, changing Ben whereas I felt awkward and clumsy. The more contact the baby can have with her father in the early weeks, the better. Given a chance, the bonding process works with fathers as well as mothers.

In some ways fathers, particularly older fathers, are more involved with their babies and children than ever before. Eighty per cent of all British fathers now attend the birth of their babies in hospital, compared with only 1 per cent ten years ago. Even when most babies used to be born at home the father would be more likely to be putting the kettle on or pacing up and down in another room than to be present at the birth. Many of the contributors to this book, especially the men themselves, said how delighted the fathers were with the baby and how much they wanted to do for them. However, they may not feel entirely sure about *what* to do. At the beginning it can be quite difficult for you to think of anyone apart from yourself and the baby, so your partner's role can be tricky. What you need most from him is support and practical help and he may not be all that used to doing the cleaning, washing, shopping, especially without being asked. You also need him to be a reassuring sounding board. But if you're like I was, you may be rather inflexible and react defensively to any criticism even if the aim is to be helpful.

The time after the birth is often strange for the partner. Clem put it this way:

> There's a huge emotional investment in the day in the labour ward. It's an amazing experience. But things had gone a bit wrong and it was a long day. All these things buzzing through your mind and you don't quite know how to make sense of it all. Then suddenly there I was, back at the house alone, after being very close, and I suppose I missed the kind of help and support that might have come from the sort of extended family *my* father had.
>
> When they came home I tended to zoom around like a dog chasing its tail, not knowing what to do for the best. I did quite crazy things like wanting to make wholesome food all the time. After Penny's complications after the birth I thought that good Geordie, north-eastern pick-me-ups would be just the thing. So there I was producing suet puddings and beef tea which Penny really didn't want and I didn't feel very appreciated.

So when I thought the nappies needed washing, he thought it would be a good idea to make elaborate meals. Perhaps disposable nappies *and* suet puddings would have been the answer, had disposables then been as good as they are now.

It is perhaps understandable, though hard for the woman to accept, that a man should want to do something creative himself at this time, rather than be the sort of support and skivvy that would be the most help. A number of women told me that their partners had inexplicably chosen the time immediately after the birth of their baby to start building a hi-fi set or decorating the living room. This sort of displacement activity seems quite funny now, looking back, but at the time it can be the core of some resentment and arguments. Perhaps you need to be much more direct about what kind of help you want. Whatever the problems of getting used to having a baby around, many fathers were actively involved in looking after their babies in the early days. What usually stopped them was *work*.

Paternity leave Provision for paternity leave in Britain is the worst in Europe. There is no state acceptance that fathers might also need time off when a baby is born and the paltry leave available to most men depends on their employer. Some men get no time at all, some two days, a few who are self-employed or have more enlightened employers can take a week or two. Most men *do* take some time off work when the baby is born but it is usually holiday which invests the time with all sorts of expectations and overtones which shouldn't apply.

In Sweden there is a total of seven months paid parental leave which can be divided between the mother and the father as they like. Up to the child's first birthday they can also work a six-hour day. In this way the state acknowledges that children are important, that bringing them up is a serious business and that parents have a right to the time to do it properly.

Work patterns If a man is in work, his thirties and forties are often an extremely demanding stage of his working life. He might not get much empathy from the people he works with – men of around his age or older may well have had their children many years before and have 'forgotten' what it's like. But the most important factor is bound to be the organization of the working day.

Most working men only see their children for a very short time each day. Having a baby might well affect his performance at work as well although perhaps being a bit older helps to get round that. Paul is 38 and a District Inspector for a Local Education Authority:

It hasn't caused me any anxieties at work but I am conscious that I'm putting less into work. What I've had to do is be much more astute about prioritizing what I do. It's been fairly calculating. I know that I'm putting in less in terms of hours, less in terms of attending meetings. What I've attempted to do is make sure that the meetings I do attend or the projects I do undertake are the ones that are going to have a larger ripple effect and, quite cynically, the ones that are going to make the greatest impression on the hierarchy.

I wasn't prepared for it at all. But I knew physically that I couldn't put in the hours because (a) I was tired and (b) it would be unfair on the kid and Sue. So very rapidly I had to make that adjustment. The initial thrust of that was survival.

It is easy to see how someone like Paul with a schedule of meetings and visits and reports, even if he does cut some out, isn't going to have a lot of time to spend with his baby. Some men don't have jobs at all but this doesn't necessarily mean that they become more involved with their children – unemployment often brings with it loss of confidence and feelings of uselessness and depression so that the man opts out of childcare too.

The men who managed to maintain their early involvement with the baby tended to be those who didn't have to bring work home with them, worked flexible hours or freelance or who deliberately altered their working lives, as women have to do, to fit in with having a child. Not surprisingly, there were very few of them. Writing in *Coming Late to Motherhood* of her experiences as a lesbian mother, Marie Ely acknowledges that her partner's flexible working hours made an enormous difference to the relationship with her child:

> My partner is a writer and a teacher and works with the flexibility of time which ensures that she is there for Susanna. Her deep commitment is separate from our relationship and is in the form of a sort of life-long guarantee. Her role, however, has a certain greyness in the eyes of society. As surrogate parent she is not mother, father, sister or even fairy godmother. There are some who would find it preferable if she did not exist, but for Susanna she provides the balance, the other half to her mother.[2]

Understanding what it's like for you It can be difficult to explain to a man who goes out to work all day what it is like to look after a small child all day every day. Andy, a haematologist, was thrilled when he and Elaine had a baby, but she felt he didn't really know what it was like: 'He still goes out to work every morning. His life has changed in that when he comes home there is me and the baby. He has no real idea of how much *my* life has changed having her.' To a man, it can seem an enviable position to be at home with the baby, something of a holiday and not at all like 'real work'. Cathy found this out very early:

> Six days after the birth John had to be away all day. He got back late at night and we were all warm and cosy. It was like an ad: here was the man coming from the big, cold outside world to this cosy little scene. And it's an absolute myth because I was absolutely exhausted with her. I hadn't even been able to make a cup of tea before midday. It was weird realizing why it's so difficult for men to know what's going on during the day. He knew enough because he'd been here all the other days, to know that it wasn't really such a cosy little scene but it's not surprising that it *appears* a dream – all snug and warm. In contrast to what he'd been doing it seemed wonderful. Whereas for me, I would have much rather been out all day, albeit at work, than dependent and stuck.

No matter how understanding and aware a particular man is, it is still generally accepted that it is the mother who will look after the baby, especially at first. She is the one who has the major adjustments to make.

Practical participation Men vary enormously in their involvement with their babies but the overall picture shows much less practical participation than the mother, whatever the circumstances, and much less than she would like, even at times when the man *is* at home, notably during weekends and holidays. A study of 75 fathers and their involvement with childcare revealed that only one in 20 thought they shared all tasks equally with the mother, especially unpleasant jobs like changing nappies.[3] Vicky:

> He did carry the baby around in a sling (she soon became too heavy for me) but he wouldn't change nappies. If he had to babysit for me, he would take off a wet nappy and leave it where it fell, but he wouldn't touch a messy one. I wonder why men think women don't mind messes and smells? Do they think they are above all that?

The fact that Vicky saw her partner as babysitting 'for' her implies that they both saw his practical role as 'helping' rather than central.

A striking number of women said that their partners won't change nappies. Interviewed by someone else, Clem said:

> I think that I've been pretty naughty. I certainly changed many more nappies in the early days, and perhaps the main problem of not being able to actually feed the baby is that you get a lot of the dirty jobs and few of the nice times. I only change nappies about four times a week now and I'm really not proud of that at all. I can't stand shitty nappies first thing in the morning.

I get very impatient with men who don't like dirty nappies – nobody likes them much, but if it's a job that has to be done, you get on with it and get used to it. The study concluded that there had been little change over the last 20 years except that more fathers these days spent more time playing with their children.

Studies of housework show that in many cases it is assumed that the woman 'manages' the household – looking after the baby and doing the housework, and that anything the man does is not really seen as his major concern but something he can offer as a favour. Tied up with this may be the recognition that being responsible for who does what (as many women seem to be) can be just as tiring as doing it yourself. Babies create an enormous amount of extra work – quite apart from the washing – other household tasks like shopping, cooking and cleaning often have to be organized in a different way.

Some women clearly don't expect much from their men and are surprisingly grateful for even a little help. Others find it inexcusable and feel much more resentful that the man's contribution should be regarded as 'help' at all rather than his share. It might be worth being very aware of the need to build on your partner's early involvement and work out with him quite specific ways of continuing his close contact. You need to be quite purposeful and strong about this and talk about it again soon if the plans don't work out. My experience bears this out as a cautionary tale. Because Clem works in television with a bar on the premises, he frequently goes there to unwind at the end of the day. I had been used to his coming home quite late and it suited me well. Little did I realize that the very time alone at the end of the day, which I had particularly enjoyed while I was working, would be the time I found Ben most difficult and needed Clem to be there. When we made plans beforehand he said the pattern would change. He would come home immediately after work he said, at 5.30 or 6 p.m., to bath the baby.

That didn't happen for much of the first year and I felt disappointed, let down and angry at Clem's lack of practical involvement with Ben. In the first few weeks he did a great deal, changing nappies and dressing Ben, walking him up and down in his restless patches. But after about six weeks he went back to his old work routine, still delighting in Ben but not so much that he wanted to do a great deal for him in that day-to-day sense. I felt very much as if I had been left holding the baby. Clem put it like this:

> For people in jobs with some stress, the interface between work and the home can be tricky. Perhaps I felt that the work day had to be diffused a little before the other role in the home – with Penny and a possibly screaming Ben – could be faced. So I would rather gravitate to a neutral place where I could wind down, with half an hour's chat and a pint, than drive through the rush hour. In the early months I really didn't know what it would be like when I got home – whether Penny would be happy and smiling or whether I would get this particular sort of half-resentful, harassed look because she might have had a bad time with Ben. I knew that even if I had to work at home, I wouldn't be able to do anything before 9 o'clock because of Ben's pattern of crying. I'm a light sleeper so I woke too in the night and there was little chance ever to catch up on sleep. I also opted out because I actually felt fairly useless. I didn't know what I could do.

Feeling left out

The disadvantage of total breastfeeding is that it is so exclusive. It is excluding of everyone except the mother but especially so of the father and I can see why some men mind about that. Breastfeeding may be a nuisance or a tie at times, especially if the baby feeds often, but it is also an incalculable pleasure. It can feel very sensuous and it is lovely to pacify a screaming baby so immediately and so personally. Perhaps men's feeling of helplessness is made worse by the fact that biologically, they can't also feed the baby themselves.

Men aren't used to being made to feel powerless and helpless by women, let alone by a baby. On the other hand, they also avoid that feeling of total responsibility the mother has of being the *only* person who can comfort a hungry, breastfed baby – a feeling both wonderful and terrible. I am sorry that I insisted on total breastfeeding for so long. It would have been good for Clem to share the pleasure of feeding and it would have been good for me to have an occasional night of unbroken sleep.

When you become the habitual comforter The ease with which you can comfort the baby on the breast can also mean that you become the habitual comforter in other ways too. Even if you don't breastfeed, the fact that you spend so much time with the baby means simply that you get to know her better. I know now that I was far too ready to intervene between Clem and Ben. For some reason I didn't think Clem should have to put up with Ben's crying, even though it upset me more than him. So if I left Ben with Clem in the house and he was restless and crying, I frequently came back and took over again. That wasn't good for any of us and leads to the 'he wants to be with you' syndrome. If I had gone out more, I wouldn't have heard him, would probably have done something more refreshing for me and he and Clem would have got more used to being together. As it was, my interference undermined their relationship and Ben became too dependent on me. This is probably one of the most important traps to look out for. Men need to have contact with their babies and to look after them in their own way, which may be different from yours.

Of course, babies cry for all sorts of reasons, not just when they're hungry and mothers become much more practised at knowing what those are. There is a definite sense of reward and achievement in being able to interpret the baby's needs so efficiently but the competence itself may be almost jealously guarded and become difficult to relinquish. So there's a double bind – you become chained to your own competence. Some women worry that if their babies spend a great deal of time with another person – whether it be a childminder, a nanny or even the father – they will lose their hold over them. It may be more sensible to be concerned about the level of *dependence* becoming too great because for some women like me, by the time you've noticed what's happening, it's too late. Angela found herself caught in a similar situation:

Tony nearly always contrived to be busy elsewhere at a change or bath time. He was prepared to baby-sit for me but his unspoken message was that it was OK for me to leave her as long as Victoria had the good manners not to soil herself or puke down his front in my absence. In her early weeks Tony seemed to look on Victoria as a live pink and white doll, interesting to watch until something good came on the television. When he spoke to her he used a strange booming tone like a department store Santa Claus which sounded very silly to me. Victoria looked uneasy when he pulled faces at her. She flinched slightly when the stubble of his beard scraped her face as he kissed her. Whatever the reason, she smiled far less often for Tony than she did for me. He noticed and reacted as if jealous. She and I were beginning to develop a close understanding while he was being left out in the cold. Although the atmosphere between Tony and myself was getting cool, I couldn't rouse enough interest in any subject outside Victoria's progress to want to talk things over. I completely lost interest in sex while I was breastfeeding and although Tony tried to understand, he felt I was rejecting him. He said that he felt almost redundant after Victoria's birth. He was merely a provider of food and shelter – no longer a lover, a companion or even a friend.

Looking back, I think I did shut him out to some extent at first. When Victoria cried so persistently in the evenings, I wanted to show off my newly acquired and hard won mothering skills. I would rush to the cot ahead of Tony, anxious to diagnose her problem quickly before she worked herself into a lather of misery. I rarely gave Tony the chance to comfort her because I honestly thought I was the only one who could 'read' her sound language.

Sharing the childcare

Whatever your intentions, it can be very difficult to share the looking after of a tiny baby. In her story in *Coming late to motherhood*, Marie Ely, a lesbian mother describes the difficulties she had with her partner who had two children of her own. Marie's baby had colic and cried a great deal:

I had talked easily and glowingly during the pregnancy about sharing the child, Not only was Susanna a child of the relationship, but we were genuinely going to divide the responsibility and decision making. But in the reality of a constantly crying child there seemed no time to talk about, let alone work through, the different perspectives we had. I found it difficult to accept the validity of my partner's experience, and to let go of gut-feelings as to what was right. Our realities spiralled off in different directions and we easily lost sight of each other. In our despair we feared the end of the relationship.

Ironically, the solution we found was a return to the traditional pattern. My partner stepped back a bit and it was agreed that I would take on the major role in Susanna's life. We resolved to begin from where I was, rather than from where I wanted to be. As a result, Susanna (like most babies) saw her mother as the centre of her universe, and related to my partner as the secondary or back-up person.[4]

Even if you don't have problems like Marie's sharing the business of looking after the baby doesn't just happen and if you don't plan for it it might not happen at all. Many fathers do look after their children on their own for a few hours or odd days but, if they are at work, that time is usually prearranged and has a finite end and they do not usually have to fit in other things as well. David:

I always enjoy looking after Jane enormously if I know I'm going to be doing it. This seems to be the distinction. For example the other day we were going out to do some shopping and Monica fell asleep. She's tired now she's pregnant again. So there I was with Jane on my hands for an indeterminate period of time and I was really annoyed. We didn't do anything constructive, just sat around, chucking a ball about, waiting for Monica to wake up which she didn't do for ages. Now I found that really bad. But if I know that I'm going to have Jane for an afternoon, I'd really enjoy it immensely. I've got the best of both worlds because when I have her it is a treat and I always do love it.

Because David doesn't look after Jane very often on a regular basis, he hasn't had to get used to the more boring things about being with a young child. It is when the childcare is not simply a 'treat' but is more equally shared that men come to understand more about what it is like.

Because they both work freelance, Bill and Helen manage to share childcare to some extent if not equally. Bill says:

> I do find it a strain if I'm looking after her for a whole day. The pattern has been that we've split in half days where possible. You realize that sometimes it's almost impossible to do anything else at the same time. In fact, I find I can actually enjoy it more if I say I can't do anything else, not even make a telephone call. Maybe the washing up – I can just about cope with that. I can understand that if you've not done it, a man can come home and say 'Look – it's a shambles – what have you been doing all day?' The idea that childcare can be *totally* demanding of your time, that's impossible to convey to someone unless they've already done it.

I remember getting home after a wonderful weekend away on my own when Clem had looked after Ben, then two and a half. A friend was coming to stay and Clem had put Ben to bed and was getting the meal ready, a meal I had half prepared before I went. 'What vegetables are we having?' I asked. 'I don't know, some from the freezer', he said. But there weren't any in the freezer. 'I haven't done any shopping; I've been looking after Ben,' he said. I couldn't resist pointing out that while I looked after Ben, I had to do other things as well.

Cathy and John do share the childcare. They both work part-time and divide up the week between them. This is very successful in fulfilling their aim of looking after Claire together but it does cause other problems. Cathy:

> We don't see each other. It's a bit of a nightmare. When you haven't got Claire, you feel you should be working so we spend very little time together as a threesome which I think is very destructive. It's like doing shift work – when one of you goes on shift the other goes off. The financial strain of both trying to earn a living in half a week is considerable. It comes back to the point that nobody pays you for looking after a kid.

Cathy's point is crucial. In most couples where the mother looks after her own child for most of the time, the man is in paid work but her work is unwaged. If she wants to return to work and the father doesn't want or can't manage to share the childcare, she has to pay someone else to look after the child. It is an important contradiction.

Making time together

Cathy mentions that she and John don't have much time together and this can be a serious strain on a relationship. Few older couples seem to resent the fact that they don't go out so much together so frequently but many mention the difference the baby makes to the kind of time they can expect. Sally:

> We were very close after he was born but I think that doesn't last. If we are together, Thomas is around and we are taking it in turns to look after him. It feels quite an occasion when we go out for a drink together and we're not actually doing something. You can slip into a position where because you're together quite a lot of the time, in the sense of being around the house and doing things with Thomas, you can not be aware that you're not spending much time together.

If you take it in turns to look after the child you can also miss out on the great pleasure there is to be had from sharing your delight in your child together. But it is very important to make time to be alone together, preferably without the baby. Try to get out regularly, say once a month. Perhaps you can get a babysitter and go out for a drink or a meal or arrange to leave the baby at a friend's house and go for a walk. Away from home it is easier to talk in a relaxed and unpressured way and even if you are sorting out difficult things, the public nature of the talk usually makes it more positive, or at least more controlled! I have found that quality of talk very necessary to a continuing understanding of each other's feelings and if we miss out on it for any length of time, we often suffer for it. We start misunderstanding each other or store up things that need to be said, sometimes leading to an explosion. Ray, Sally's partner, says something similar:

> I think there is a danger that you tend to relate through your child. It just covers up problems and feelings – what you really want to do is directly relate one to one. The child can get in the way of your own relationship. You have to try to preserve what is the sharing between you and the child that you have and that part of your life which is the relationship with the other person. It's very difficult to maintain that balance.

Acknowledging the strain

There are some things that are very complex to talk about at all, as Kay found:

It's only now (after four months) that he's accepting the fact that he's got a son, he's a father. It's taken him a long time. He didn't like what I was becoming. He couldn't handle that and he couldn't handle this little mite suddenly disrupting his whole life. He'd come in and this baby was still there at midnight demanding my attention and we couldn't have a conversation. I started to resent his lack of involvement after a while because I thought he was almost saying, 'Well, you wanted a baby, didn't you? I've done my bit. You've got a nice, healthy son, now get on with it.' That was amazing because before he was full of, 'Let's share parenthood. I'll do this and I'll adjust to that.' I was more keen if I was going to have someone to help me. He actually said yesterday that he was really pleased he'd got a son. That was a relief! In fact, we went through quite a sticky patch. I'd even thought maybe it wasn't going to survive. He was going one way and I was going another. We weren't even talking to each other anymore. And I thought, I'm not going to live like this. There was a lot of stress in the relationship. You'd think after nine years there'd be a lot of strength in it, but this little fellow really put it to the test. I wish I'd known a bit more about how a man might or might not cope, even a man you think you know well. If I'd done a bit more thinking about that I wouldn't have been so hurt and switched off because I thought, I can't cope with *him*. I'm just going to concentrate on me and the baby, which was a shame really because I'm sure it shut Steve out. Now I've come round, we're getting on much better.

I felt a bit cold towards him because I felt he wasn't doing his bit. I never regretted having Adam. It was more, why should I make allowances for Steve? I'm going very carefully. I can't be pushy and intense about it because he just switches off. I don't want to alienate him from his son.

When I asked Kay whether she thought Steve would be prepared to talk to me, she laughed and said 'chance would be a fine thing'. Only a handful of men accepted the invitation made through over 100 women volunteers to talk or write about their experiences. 'He doesn't like expressing personal feelings' was a typical response.

Ten men agreed to a taped interview and three or four wrote about their views. Since I know some of the contributors I asked some men directly whether they would take part. The reaction was often unease, a blank face, a mutter about having nothing interesting to say, occasionally a more overt disinclination to discuss anything so personal. I was surprised and disappointed by this although I am well aware that there is a difference between the way most men and most women talk about personal experience and possibly the way they think about it too. The intimacy that women have with each other is probably quite rare in men.

The way society is organized means that it is often expected that not only will men normally be in control but they will also be controlled about their deepest feelings. They are not used to expressing doubts or fears or questioning themselves out loud to anyone not extremely close to them or perhaps at all. David finds little chance to talk about his deep feelings for his daughter:

> I do talk about her at work but it's not done in a straight way. It's a bit jokey. I feel slightly annoyed that of all the people I know who've got children, only one bloke has ever said anything with feeling about his child. I've actually said to people, 'Why didn't you tell me it was so fantastic?'

Men miss out on the kind of supportive talk that women have much more easily. It is possible for women to talk openly about problems without feeling threatened by admitting to them – the network of support that is the core of the Women's Movement.

Having a baby can sometimes separate you from the friends you used to talk to, especially if they don't have children and don't share your new absorbing interest. You also have less time available to your friends, especially child-free time and occasions like simply going out for a drink become much harder to organize. Some people find it almost impossible to see established friends on the same basis, as Bill says:

> I have come very close to losing male friendships. My closest friend I used to see two or three times a week. I now see him maybe every three weeks. He's become a father at the same time. I think if either of us had not had children almost

simultaneously we would have been quite hurt by that and I do miss the friendship I had. Maybe some of the things I would have talked about with him I now talk about with Helen more. I don't think that's necessarily a good thing. The idea of concentrating everything on one relationship puts on a weight that it can't quite take.

Sex

Talk isn't the only way of expressing your feelings. A physical and sexual relationship also matters a great deal and for many people this changes quite dramatically for a time after the birth. Susan:

> Just having had a baby, we had no physical relationship. Perhaps in the past if we couldn't sort things out by sitting down and talking about it, we would eventually on those occasions when we made love. We had no relationship like that to cover it, so that probably made it worse. I couldn't cope with the physical side. And the old-fashioned guilt feeling – a man wants it more than a woman. It's a psychological thing. You probably are physically all right but it's getting over that first time.

It can be almost intimidating to be told to wait six weeks after the birth before intercourse, as if you should expect problems. Yet I found making love painful or uncomfortable for nearly six months, for 'psychological' reasons I was told by male doctors. It is quite common to feel some discomfort for a considerable time, especially after an episiotomy. Breastfeeding can affect the natural lubrication of the vagina and the vagina can also feel dry if you take the mini pill (the progestogen-only pill). If your breasts or nipples are sore, or spout milk the moment they are touched, that can be off-putting too; so is having to wear a bra at night for support. In other societies people often abstain from sex for specific periods after a birth, and usually longer than the six weeks advised in Britain. It may be a good idea to talk about it with your partner and set a certain limit when you won't have sex (whether for a short or long period). Then you can start negotiating once that time is over. It's nice to have an agreed period when you don't have to think about it if you don't want to.

At least having a physical reason for not enjoying sex is an explanation or excuse for going off the idea. You could also find that there just isn't enough of the right kind of time for making love once you have a baby. You go to bed at different times perhaps and when you do get to bed the only thing you really want to do is sleep. There is usually little chance of waking up in the morning before the baby does. Rosalind: 'We've missed the lack of privacy; one doesn't imagine a tiny baby can put such a stop to one's sex life. One is either too tired or the baby needs feeding, changing, winding, etc. I think it has been worse for my husband than for me, because I wanted the baby more than he did.' Exhaustion is probably the greatest interference factor. Although making love might well increase your sense of wellbeing afterwards, getting round to doing it can be difficult. You might not feel much like your old self anyway. Diane:

> It was the situation in the evenings which had the most disastrous effect on us. I felt totally frustrated that there never seemed to be time to do anything – write letters, read, sew or forget about being a mother first, last and foremost! I felt drained and lacking in any feeling of self (hard to explain, but there was no time when I could be me and do what I wanted to do). We didn't seem to draw together. I felt tense, guilty (as though it was my fault) and my overwhelming desire was to be left alone. It certainly wasn't encouraging for a happy relationship. Basically, if you never know when you'll be interrupted but are sure that interruptions will occur, you lose heart about any physical relationship. Besides, it all seems terribly irrelevant anyway.

One man said that he found the idea of possible interruptions rather exciting but I don't think that is many people's experience. A number of women say they felt guilty about their changed attitude to physical or sexual contact. Janice:

> I found it very hard to give my husband enough physical contact. In some ways we were living in parallel not in contact. Poor man, that really continued for five years because of the subsequent little ones and the constant demand for physical touching was more than I could supply. I sometimes felt that I'd scream if another child or person got hold of me.

The feeling that Janice describes of not wanting to be touched, of wanting to be left alone, is very familiar to me, especially at the end of the day after Ben's gone to bed. It must seem hard to Clem because the end of his working day is just the time he wants cuddles. He doesn't get the same physical contact that I do during the day. I remember being surprised some years ago when a friend said that she wasn't interested in sex anymore, because her young children were so sexy. She didn't need more than that. I understand that now that I know more about the warmth and snuggliness of babies and small children. The holding and hugging and cuddling is lovely but it may also fulfil much of the need for physical contact. And because women get so much more of that, it isn't surprising that some men feel sexually rejected.

While you can't force yourself to make love if you don't want to, there may be other ways of getting some of the closeness and intimacy that sex gives. Angela found that after the initial strain, things improved, especially after Victoria was fully weaned from the breast at a year old:

> My milk dried up quickly and I began to feel more independent and energetic, more myself and less of a walking lunch counter. I bought some new dresses and joined a keep-fit class to tone up my still flabby muscles. As my appearance improved, my desire for sex gradually returned and it became easier to talk to Tony once we were in close physical contact again. We talked for hours in bed, wrapped in the privacy of darkness and quiet. I began to see that all the while I wanted him to take turns putting nappies through the wash and buttoning up babygros, he was trying to build up a new business which could give us financial security in the future, He would drive home from work dog-tired from humping heavy machinery with only a few hours broken sleep in prospect. What matters to me now is that he supported me in his way as well as he understood how. If we had communicated better I could have enabled him to do more. In the end having a baby strengthened our marriage. As parents we came face to face with each other as people. Through loving her we have come to enjoy a deeper appreciation of each other's powers and limits, fears and dreams.

There are many adjustments you will make with your partner once you have a baby. Shona:

> In retrospect I see that the adjustments need to be gradual and

you cannot expect overnight parenthood even though it's expected of you. In saying I need John more now, I mean that I feel I have so much to do with Timmy that I need someone to think about me. I often worry about doing the right thing and need feedback from time to time that I'm being OK at mothering and that my child is receiving all the attention and stimulation he should be. But to do that, I feel that I need my own confidence boosting and my own ego pampered – and it does not always happen! Previously I suppose I gained satisfaction and personal fulfilment from my job. Now I get most of it from my family and probably more from my son than my husband! I think that if you are to constantly 'give' to a child (and the first year is mostly giving), you need to be 'given' a bit in return from a partner.

It is not just affection or caring but the feeling that you *matter* that needs to be conveyed. Otherwise you end up feeling a bit like an empty tank. It has taken me some time to get this into words for John but I think he now has the message and whether or not I receive my quota of attention now depends not on lack of understanding but on pressure of work or finance which are less threatening reasons.

Shona has clearly had to work hard to get John to see things from her point of view – the differing perspectives are complex to explain and often lead to misunderstanding but it's good to pursue them and try to work them out.

The pleasures you share

This chapter, like some of the others, has focused on the difficulties you and your partner may face in settling down to being first-time parents in your thirties and forties. Up to now it looks as if it's all problems and of course that's ridiculous. Alongside any stresses and strains is a huge base of shared pleasure and enrichment, the kind of feeling that prompts Sue to say:

I don't think anyone can ever top that, just having a child together. I think there's nothing that can bring you closer than that. Things that happen afterwards could take you farther away again – all the tension and strain – but there's a cord that holds you together. We have a really good laugh now. (William is just a year). He's lovely – the greatest thing you

could have. Whenever we feel fed up we just have to go and
look at him but I don't think it's something I'd have
appreciated when I was younger. He has a joke with you and
he giggles and giggles. We don't know what the joke is but
something makes him laugh. If we didn't smile he wouldn't be
giggling. I don't know what's going on in his mind that he
finds so funny but he sits there like a little old man going ho,
ho, ho.

Paul also really values William's entertainment value:

There's no reason why he suddenly hits himself on the head
but he does and it's very entertaining. I change him, I bath
him, I feed him, I do everything that has to be done. It's an
absolute hoot. That's part of the fun because it's tremendously
messy and tremendously uninhibited.

But those intense feelings are very private. As Paul said on
p. 122, you don't share them with other people because you think
they would be bored. And they would. But because it isn't
appropriate to dwell on the joy and also because it is partly
indescribable, don't forget that it's there.

Everyone comments on how their life together has been
enriched by the baby. Here is Philip:

It has been much more fun that I thought it would be and as a
joint venture has brought us closer together rather than
divided us. A good deal has been written about how
motherhood involves enormous changes, especially for ex-
working mothers (that's not intended to be a sexist remark – I
do not imply that motherhood is not work – it is just unpaid).
Less has been said about the changes involved in being a
father. These are rather subtle, to do with outlook and it is
difficult to be concrete about them. I think for both of us it has
added another dimension, perhaps like seeing in 3D rather
than 2D or hearing in stereo rather than mono.

People talk with pleasure of doing things together with their
child that they might not have done at all – going to a street fair
or for a walk in the country or to the zoo. Being with a small child
is fun and gives you the excuse to fool around in ways long
forgotten – that kind of unselfconsciousness is quite rejuvenating.
Colin:

I do the shopping with Joe. He goes out with me on Saturday morning and if the weather's good as well I carry him in the back pack. It's very nice and we plod off on a much longer route than I need to do and it's a nice walk and he loves it. You can't get closer than having a baby on your back. It's smashing to have Joe catching hold of my ears – the number of people it cheers up to see him. He bounces back and forward. I couldn't imagine that a child could bring so much pleasure in ten months. He's such a healthy and happy child. He sucks up enjoyment and blows it out again.

Having a small child also gives you the chance to do things you'd like to do anyway, like having a ride on a steam train or sunbathing in the garden with your feet in the paddling pool. And simply because there is no one else in the world who has an equally deep investment in the child, you *can* go on talking about your child with your partner. Reliving it by talking about it is an extra pleasure and it all brings about a closeness that is very special.

9

On your Own: Being a Single Parent

Heather had been living with her partner for four and a half years when they decided to have a baby. It took her a year and a half to conceive and when she was four months pregnant, Ian left her very suddenly for a much younger woman whom she later married. Since then she has been on her own.

I'd never seen myself as the maternal type but I was over 30 when it first occurred to me that if I didn't soon have any children I would no longer have the choice. It's the old biological clock. Men don't have this problem, women do. We decided it would be a good time – all our friends were having babies. There would be support, mutual experiences to share, no financial difficulties. He was the best planned baby ever.

One of the ironic reasons for having a baby was because I knew Ian would be a very good father – children really get on well with him. It seems very hard to say that now seeing that he's not come near our child for such a long time.

It was very sudden. I switched from being a 'wife' to being a mother. I never became a wife *and* a mother. One minute I had a husband in effect, the next minute I had a child. It was a very, very drastic change. There I was overnight, with responsibilities, and it was a fantastic shock.

One in eight families in Britain have only one parent and by far the greatest number of these are mothers. Although the number of single parents is increasing, social attitudes change less quickly and it is not easy to be the only parent in a society that still largely organizes itself around couples. The women who contributed to this chapter are not representative of all single parents – there are too few of them for that. For example, some mothers don't live with a partner and have the main responsibility for their children, but do live with other adults. Some women, like Heather, become single parents by default and for many others, the relationship with their partner breaks up after their babies (or children) are born.

However there are women, particularly those over 30, who decide that they would rather be single parents than risk not having a baby at all. The urge to have a baby can be very strong. On p. 6. Marian describes how she planned her baby quite deliberately over some years knowing she would be on her own. Writing later about her experiences as a single parent in an article in *The Chartist*, Marian goes on:

> I am very proud of being a deviation, but I could not possibly recommend it as a course of action to any but the most committed, with a plentiful reserve of energy, patience, ingenuity, and access to an acceptable level of material comforts. In the first year of my son's life I was at home with him and had only him for company 24 hours a day – it certainly felt like that while he was breastfed and waking all through the night. They say the relationship between a first baby and its mother is akin to a love affair – I'd agree – every little action is a delight – but it palls, if that's all the action there is. And without a sense of proportion and a measure of what some might call maturity, this is the stage when resentment can start, and with the relentless day and night demands of the totally self-centred infant, it becomes easier and easier to allow yourself to express that resentment in rough handling of the baby. Unchecked, this, as we all know, leads to child abuse. It can happen in two-parent families where the load is not shared, but it's a lot more likely when there is no other adult to share the aggravation.[1]

Marian chose to have her baby and although life is difficult she would not have it otherwise. Nor would Alice who had no intention at all of having baby at that stage of her life. She was a mature student in her second year of a degree course when she became pregnant during a relationship with a man who was studying in England for a year and had to return to South America. After the initial shock she was quite pleased to be pregnant but was horrified by the way she was treated at the hospital where she was to have her baby. Being a student and being black meant that insulting assumptions were made about her:

> My initial contact with the hospital was 'you're a loose woman, it's got to be a one-night stand'. They just couldn't see that you could be going out with someone seriously even though it was for a short time. It wasn't permanent and I knew that from the beginning. They put 'social problem' in my records. I thought they themselves had a problem because in no way do I see myself as a social problem. I thought if that is their attitude then I'm not surprised that young people are not going to turn up to their clinic. I reckon that at my age what right have they to tell me I'm a loose woman, having gone through life right up to 30 without a child. It's their lack of sensitivity and imagination – I don't think women should have that attitude to other women.
>
> When I was leaving the hospital, they said – 'all right – see you next year'. So it was a matter of: you're a loose woman anyway but before next year you'll be back with another one-night stand. The whole attitude was so wrong. They'd actually appointed a social worker for me without knowing my circumstances. And I thought well, we'll see who is most positive. I felt that OK, I've had the child, there was no way I was going to give it up. I didn't consider an abortion.

Yvonne did consider having an abortion when she became pregnant at the age of 30. In fact, she got as far as having the pre-med and going down to the operating theatre before she decided not to go through with it. She had been living with her baby's father on and off for 13 years but by the time she knew she was pregnant he had gone to India where he was becoming very involved in a religious community (see chapter 1, p. 8).

Being on your own as the better alternative

Comparatively few women start out as single mothers like Heather, Alice and Yvonne. It is more common for babies to be born to two parents living together, the breaking up of their relationship coming some time later. Rising divorce figures show that fewer people now 'stay together for the sake of the children'. Although the break-up of a relationship is always painful, emotionally upsetting and exhausting, it can be a much happier alternative than struggling on in an uncomfortable, acrimonious or miserable partnership. Paula had her baby with the tacit approval of her partner although he showed little enthusiasm and did not help her at all with the baby, even though she went back to a full-time teaching job when Christopher was four and a half months old.

Finally, after I had been too exhausted to have sex with him one night he decided I must be having an affair with somebody else (no comment) and a few days later beat me up very brutally. If the baby had not finally woken up terrified by my screams and started screaming also (I shall never forget his screams of terror) I do not know what would have happened. Somehow I managed to get the baby out of the flat and fled to some people I know nearby, and called the police.

When I made it clear that under no circumstances would I consider going back to him, he stopped coming to see the baby. To me this was a great relief. He had beaten me up on three previous occasions and when I think about my life with him now I wonder at myself. I do not feel bitter about it, however, as I have my darling little boy, and would much rather go it alone than be tied to this man, who was so possessive that I could not have friends or life of my own at all. I've never regretted my decision to break free from him (I had been trying to get him to agree to a separation before all this happened) and when people say to me, 'The baby must tie you down,' I think secretly, 'Not half as much as his father did.'

If you are living in the sort of tense atmosphere that Paula describes, being on your own, even as a single parent, has to be an improvement. Helena separated from her husband under similarly violent circumstances after struggling to cope with his growing mental illness for well over a year. When he was finally persuaded to leave, her baby was ten months old and her life changed radically.

I was able to go out in the evenings. While he was here he wouldn't go out. Occasionally we would go out together, with Josh, because he would never have anyone in to babysit. He'd never have anyone in the house at all. I managed to get babysitters and started going to yoga and seeing people again. Friends started coming round here. Because James was so difficult they had stopped coming round. He always thought I was going to see lovers. It was much better for Josh – his lifestyle improved because he was able to have contact with other people.

Help and support

Having contact with other people improved Helena's life too. If you live on your own it can be a very frightening prospect to be entirely responsible for looking after your baby. Especially at the beginning it can be very hard, if you have no way of handing the baby over to someone else. Rather like starting a demanding and completely different new job, not feeling 100 per cent well, on half the normal amount of sleep, getting no pay and having no one on tap to give you advice or cheer you up. Here is Marian:

> The total chaos was very unsettling. The sense of continual crisis – not in handling of the baby, he and I were in perfect tune – but in the supporting practical tasks: organizing the washing, attempting to feed myself, keeping a track of mail, phone calls. Always having to answer the door with my blouse undone (constant breastfeeding!!). Trying to cope with one of the cats being very demanding, upset and jealous. Never sleeping more than three hours, often less, never feeling able to relax – feeling at the mercy of the tiny babe – life and body not your own. I didn't feel in the slightest resentful of his demands, I just could scarcely keep up. My sister stayed with me for the first week, then I was on my own. I've been on my own ever since. The panic didn't really let up for months.

Heather was frightened to leave the hospital to go home, partly because the baby had jaundice quite badly:

> I didn't like being in hospital but I was terrified of going home with a possibly sick baby on my own. I asked my mother if she would come and stay with me and she did – she stayed for a total of three weeks. My mum's nearly 70 and I felt guilty asking her to stay for such a long time but I'm glad she did.

Her mother was probably glad to be able to help even if she was pleased to return to her own house.

As has been said in countless places elsewhere in this book, *all* mothers need support and help. But single mothers especially need a break, a shoulder, and some practical help. You have to find ways of asking for help that actually convey the need and Yvonne found that that can be very difficult:

> It was really hard trying to tell people. Saying to people as bluntly as I could – I need help, I'm not coping, I'm just on the knife-edge and I could fall over at any time. But because I gave the *appearance* of coping very well what I got from people was assurance that I *was* coping very well. I had the feeling sometimes that it was like talking in a foreign language, that you actually knew the vocabulary but you didn't know the nuances and the colloquial expressions. I'd be saying this and they just wouldn't understand what I was saying. They'd say: but obviously it's great. Your work's good, you're getting it in on time, the baby's thriving – *you* look pretty healthy. Not *hearing* what I was saying and I was saying it as bluntly as I could. I wasn't hinting at it. They were people who had no children.

People who don't have any children often don't know what it's like and even those who do, forget. You have to tell them. And that means being quite specific about what would help. You need to be able to ring someone up on a miserable Sunday and say, 'Look, this baby is driving me mad – please come and see us or take her out for a bit.' If people offer to babysit for you, let them. If they invite you round for a meal, go, even if it seems all too much trouble to arrange. If people ask if they can help, say yes and tell them what they can do. You may feel guilty at times but think how good they'll feel! Adults also get a lot out of being with children.

Feeling alone

Even if you are lucky enough to get offers of help and are self-protective enough to use them fruitfully, or if you are also surrounded by people who want to have a relationship with your child, in the end you are the one person responsible for your baby and that can make you feel very alone. Not only is there no one to care about you and to put back some of the love and mental energy you expend on your child, but there is no one to share the other things that go with looking after a child. Marian:

The other side of this adult isolation is that there is also no one there to share the joys – the charming antics, the sweet expressions and quaint attempts at speech. No one to share immediately the triumph of the baby's mastery of the physical world. So while bearing and nurturing a child have been, to me, deeply emotionally satisfying, there it stops. Without a supportive and admiring circle of friends and relatives, the pleasure and the pain is all yours.

Writing two years later, things hadn't improved much for Marian in that personal sense:

I often feel we are totally outside organized family society and are not considered part of the single world either. Daniel and I live in a limbo with each other. You can imagine that weekends are not good and now I dread and hate Christmas. People have been asking what do you want for Christmas, and I have to say I really don't need anything – except a loving partner, and of course money doesn't buy one of those.

It is easy to imagine that everybody is having a much nicer time than you are, especially at times of enforced holiday and commercialized jollity like Christmas when it feels particularly lonely to be on your own. Weekends too can be hard, not just for single mothers but also for women whose partners do not share much of the childcare. Yvonne has found that too:

There's an expectation that weekends are supposed to be lovely and everyone's out enjoying themselves. It's very often a lot easier to cope with half a dozen kids under six than just one because they'll amuse each other. So often, if I couldn't off-load Sam on to somebody I'd have their kids in, thus giving the impression that I was being ever so generous but in fact there was a pay-off for me.

Another strategy Yvonne developed has been to let Sam stay up later than usual on a Friday night so that he will sleep later the next morning and give her some extra time in bed. She also found that he loved going to big supermarkets and riding in the trolley so she does a monthly shop which is a treat for him and useful for her. This sort of self-interested analysis of how to make life easier for yourself is important for all mothers but can be a lifeline for a single parent.

The father's place

Many women worry about how their babies will feel about not having a father around, especially those children who rarely or never see their fathers. Helena: 'I wonder how Josh is going to react when he's older to not having a father around. He's got pictures of James on the wall and he knows it's daddy and that daddy's in Durham. But I wonder what stage he's going to wonder *why* daddy is in Durham. I worry about that a bit.' It is possible for some children to continue seeing their fathers on a regular basis but that is often difficult for the mother, especially since when they are small it may be more convenient for the father to come and visit the child in her own environment. That isn't easy for the man either and sometimes it simply becomes too painful to continue. Whatever your hopes for maintaining the relationship it doesn't always work out. Vaughan Melzer is a lesbian mother who described her experiences in *Coming Late to Motherhood*:

> When I set out to have my baby, I saw myself as a single parent with the loving and emotional support of my friend and lover and, to some extent, the baby's father. How these relationships were to be in practice was not initially clear. Carole came to live with me and, in this, I am not a single parent though, in the eyes of the conventional world, I am. This results in some social discomfort at times but also in practical benefits (for example, if Carole were my husband I would not be eligible for a nursery place).
>
> Billy's father visits about once a month, viewing his relationship with Billy as an avuncular one. This relationship, though warm and affectionate, does have its problems. I could not have made a baby with just anyone: the father had to be someone I respected and admired and for whom I felt affection. He reciprocates these feelings, and inevitably there is some pain that for our individual reasons we have not got a conventional marriage together.[2]

A year later she added an afterword:

> Well, over a year has passed and my situation has changed a lot. Some months ago, by mutual but painful consent, Carole and I separated. Despite the pleasure I experienced in the

constant sharing and companionship, I did not feel ready to share my life and I felt a great sense of relief to be living independently once again. At the same time Billy's father decided he could not cope with the situation and we now have no contact with him. So the two people who influenced and assisted me so significantly in having my child are both uninvolved at the moment.[3]

Yvonne discovered that she was pregnant when her baby's father, Ron, had gone to India after a lengthy but fluctuating relationship. Ron was involved with Sam immediately after his birth but for the next three years saw very little of him. As Sam has got older and his father's circumstances have changed, they have spent more time together although Yvonne and Ron don't have the same kind of relationship that they had before. This has some advantages for Yvonne who actually managed to leave Sam with his father for a week when he was four and have a holiday in Spain on her own. 'That was terrific – a smashing present.'

In some ways it may be easier to know that you are not going to see your baby's father at all and to avoid the disruption and churning emotions of occasional visits. The father of Alice's child is in Mexico and although he knows that they have a child, they are no longer in contact. Alice has, however, talked about her daughter's father since Maria was very young.

> At the nursery she came home and she was near to tears – she was saying that everybody else has got a father and I haven't. And I said, that's not quite how it goes. Everybody's got a father but they don't necessarily live with their mothers and their child. I think it does help if you tell them reasonably early. And if you're reasonably honest, there are a lot of advantages. I don't feel that a myth should develop about him.

Marian feels uneasy about Daniel's growing awareness – writing when he is four and a half she says:

> It wasn't until September this year that he asked about 'daddy' and is now aware of the absence of a dad here. His behaviour I think reflects this and you can imagine I feel somewhat awkward about this as I conceived him on purpose knowing there'd be no dad. Sometimes I wonder what I started and whether I can stop the mad roundabout of skewed development that seems to be inevitable.

It can be quite salutary to remember that having a father around all the time might create its own difficulties. Heather:

> I know deep down that if Tom's dad was still with us there would be major conflicts about the way we brought him up. That might have created problems. By and large I think children should have more than one adult to relate to – it doesn't matter if it's the father. It could be the mother and friends, it could be the father and friends. I don't think one adult is enough and this is a thing that gets me down.

Perhaps one way of dealing with the absence of a father is to set out quite deliberately to spend time with other adults and get to know other single-parent families, so that your child grows up with families that have one parent as well as those that have two. Helena has made this an important part of her dealings with Josh since James left and since she has a big enough house, she also has two other adults living there as lodgers, which gives Josh other adults to relate to and provides built-in babysitting. Sharing a house with other adults who like children does seem to be a very happy way round some of the problems of isolation, quite apart from its obvious usefulness.

Relationships with other men

As a single mother another fragile area is the kind of relationships you can make with other men. Several women talk about their unease both about having sufficient opportunity to meet other men and then, if they do, the strains that being a mother places on any developing relationship. Heather goes out with someone who works at her office:

> I wouldn't have met him if he didn't work there. I don't go anywhere to meet people. The relationship is singularly one-sided because I am available whenever he wants to come and see me but he is never available when I want to see him. It seems to reinforce the old sexual stereotypes. The man decides when we're going to go out, where we're going to go, what we're going to do and that has to be set up in advance. It's not a very satisfactory relationship. If I were more able to go out and meet other groups of people and do other things then the chances are I'd have packed it in a long time ago. But I'm

actually quite afraid of having no one at all, at my age, if I'm honest about it. It's sort of morally wrong because I feel as if *I'm* using him as well.

Heather's friend doesn't know many children and finds it hard to relate well to Tom. Furthermore it was becoming clear that Tom didn't like him which made things very difficult for her. Possibly it's even worse though, if your child does form a strong attachment to a man in your life as happened to Marian:

> It took me 18 months to miss having a relationship with a man and I have made all sorts of efforts ever since. I had a marvellous friend from August 1983 to very recently, but that has now gone down the drain and Daniel and I feel the loss very greatly. We both became very fond of him and this is such a problem, exploring and establishing a relationship when there is a child around. You can no longer afford to be casual, but it puts too great a strain on a new relationship to insist upon the commitment necessary because of the expectations and needs of the child. One does get so badly out of practice of talking intimately to anyone having this sort of isolated life.

The bonuses

Although it is clearly an exhausting and difficult job to bring up your child on your own, there are some aspects of that life that may be enviable. Because they have had more experience and have a sharper realization that everything *isn't* so rosy for everybody else, women over 30 who are single parents often value their special advantages. For example, Helena tells of a morning when she went to drop Josh off on her way to work at the house of the friend with whom she shares a nanny. She and her husband were both there:

> Mark's away quite a lot of the time but this particular day they were both together in the morning and he was obviously late for work. He was saying, '*Where's* my button?' and 'Why isn't this and what about that?' and I was thinking – well, it's really very nice. I don't have any of that hassle. It's the feeling that I only have Josh to relate to, not another person as well. If Josh and I want to do something we can go off and do it and don't have to think whether the other person wants to do it. That's quite nice.

Men can take a fair bit of looking after as well as children. Even if a partner doesn't always expect a meal on the table when he comes in from work (and a lot of men still do), men do create a great deal of extra housework. So it can be good not having to think about that. Single mothers also value the fact that there aren't two sets of rules in the house, two views about how to bring the child up, and feel that much conflict is avoided because of that.

For Alice, having a child and having to cope on her own has been extremely positive and she feels she has grown in confidence and maturity by being forced back on her own resources:

> When I was younger I was very scatty. I just didn't know the meaning of being responsible. I think it's helped me to think out what I really do want and what I don't want. I've had such a full life I don't feel deprived having to stay at home if I can't find a babysitter. As far as possible, rather than looking at it as something negative that stopped me doing *a, b* and *c*, I think of it as a positive thing that's going to help me carry on and help me to plan my life and the child's life. Things that I worry about now didn't worry me before. If I didn't pay a month's rent I wouldn't worry about it but now I do, and think next thing they'll have the bailiffs out after me. Because I've got this tendency to be slightly eccentric at times, I felt that I needed something to bring me back to reality.

Valerie thinks she copes better now than she would have done when she was younger. She lives alone with Mark but has a close relationship with his father and sees him regularly. He is married to someone else with other children so cannot spend much time with them. At times it has been very hard, especially since Mark was a very bad sleeper and when Val has been ill.

> I think I've got a bit more patience than I would have had ten years ago, certainly more sense. I don't think I could have coped with the same situation ten years ago. Living the way I have has made me so independent that it's made life a lot easier to cope with. At times I felt I was going round the bend. I think ten years ago I *would* have gone round the bend.

Now that her daughter is getting older (she is four and a half) Alice is getting more and more out of her:

When I get her something new she really appreciates it. She says, 'Good girl, Alice. That is really nice of you and I'm going to listen to you from now on.' It's really quite a lovely relationship. If I was on my own I wouldn't know about things like that. It's a new learning experience for me and it's something special.

Yvonne has found that her life too has been enriched by Sam:

I can still think that rationally I made the wrong decision but I don't regret that I took the wrong decision at all. I've enjoyed it and I get an awful lot of satisfaction out of Sam. I had a very happy childhood and I think one reason perhaps why you want children yourself is so you can relive it. I play the same games with him as my mother played with me. You can go through the whole process again only somebody else is the child.

Looking after yourself

If you are on your own you are looking after your child but no one is looking after you. It takes a pretty determined effort and a deliberate sense of self-interest to look after yourself. This might be on a pretty basic level – like seeing that you eat properly. Yvonne found that once she went back to work, having a slow cooker made a huge difference:

If I got up early I could put a meal on and then take Sam to the day nursery. By the time I got home at about 6 o'clock, there was no business about having to set to and cook. You took the lid off and there was your evening meal. That was terrific because if I didn't do that, I'd come home tired and I wouldn't cook. And if I didn't eat it just spiralled. For somebody on their own some method of getting good food into you quickly is invaluable – a deep freeze or microwave oven could do the same, I suppose.

Women, who often make great efforts to cook for other people, rarely feel it is important to cook for themselves. Eating healthily might be one of the things that go for a single mother but it can be very dispiriting to find that you eat snacks all the time and it is worth finding some alternative.

Eating isn't the only way of feeding yourself. You need also to do things that are just for you, that you will enjoy and that perhaps have nothing to do with your baby or your job. Yvonne makes time for some things but not others:

> I'd pull out the stops and make an effort for a night at the Opera. I wouldn't make an effort to go down to the local and have a couple of jars. That kind of thing went. If you've got to set up the babysitting arrangements you've got to set them up for something that is really worth doing. There was a change in my life but it didn't hurt much. But if you're a single parent and you're gregarious it must be very hard to be tied to the house in the evening.

Heather would like to have a much more sociable life than she does but finds it difficult to get out to do the things she would like to do. Being tied down at home has affected her confidence since she has always tended to be shy anyway:

> It can be too much trouble to arrange babysitting. If you are feeling hesitant about whether you can face going to see a group of intelligent people and discuss things other than child-rearing with them, you will make excuses not to go. I haven't read a good book since before I had Tom (two and a half years ago). I've got folded up bits of *The Guardian* lying around that I intend to read and I never get round to reading them. I'm a member of the Labour Party. I've never been to a meeting. I wouldn't dare go. There's a *Women's* section but I'm frightened of going. I might have to say something. I might reveal my ignorance – the fact that I've been cut off from the outside world as it were. My confidence has been eroded – I'm a lot less confident than I was.

It is easy to understand why Heather feels like that even though she handles her job as a Senior Housing Officer perfectly competently. It is at a personal level that she has lost faith and although one can stand outside all that and say it wouldn't be nearly as bad as she thinks if she *did* go to a Labour Party meeting, she probably needs someone to go with, the first time at least. Looking after yourself may mean asking people to share those things with you, difficult as that may be.

Babysitting can be a real problem if you're a single parent, especially if you cannot afford to pay for it. A babysitting circle might not help much because your ability to babysit for other people is very limited. Some organized groups do offer babysitters but it takes time to build up a group of people you can rely on and whom your baby will trust too.

Getting a living

Single mothers either have to work or live off the state. There is no alternative. For this reason, many single mothers over 30 do go back to work and find that working not only earns the money they need but also offers important companionship and status. The issues that affect working mothers are covered in detail in chapter 11 and they all apply, if in a more stretching way, to single mothers. Heather felt relieved in some way that she had no option about working: 'One advantage of being a single parent is that I've never had to worry about whether it is better for me to be at home looking after my child myself or whether it is better to be at work.' Of the single mothers I talked to, only Valerie had chosen not to work:

> I've always worked – as a telephonist, receptionist. Before that I was at a tobacco factory, before that hairdressing. I don't know how I found time to go to work. I don't have the money I did have. I'm on Social Security which is hardly enough to manage. My mum's a great help to me – she runs the car. But it has been a strain. I've no intention of going to work until he goes to school and even then it'll only be work inside his school hours. My mother never worked. I think a mother's place is with her child and I'm quite happy to spend all my time with him. He's my first concern.

It is extremely difficult to live on Social Security, not simply because it is so little money but also because of the cumbersome and humiliating bureaucratic procedures that are part and parcel of claiming Supplementary Benefit. If you have had several years as an independent adult, earning your own living, this is very hard to take. Marian took extended maternity leave and lived on Social Security so she could spend the first year of Daniel's life with him, but she found it a shock to be so poor: 'I'm slowly adjusting to poverty. It's never happened to me before but I never look round the shops because I've got no money. Never do window shopping anymore. Christmas was a nightmare – I got round it by going to White Elephant stalls at jumble sales.'

For Alice, things were also very hard in the first year after her baby was born, while she was unemployed. She had given up the degree course she was taking and couldn't find a job:

> If you're an older woman with kids, at the back of your mind you think, well really, at this age, should I be going to the DHSS saying look I need more money? You'd prefer to suffer it. There were times when I'd actually go to my mother every single day to eat because I didn't have the money to look after the child. I had big electricity bills – the flat was all electric and she was two months old in winter. Whatever remained couldn't pay the rent, rates and water rates. There was nothing left out of forty pounds a week Supplementary Benefit for food. At that point I was at my lowest. I thought – I've got this child. It doesn't matter about me but how am I going to feed her? So I'd go to my mother's. I'd just sit there and look at her and she'd know that I was really hitting rock bottom. She had retired and her income was thirty-four pounds a week which didn't help matters at all.

It is clear that a single mother managing on her own depends on her relatives and friends not only for practical help but sometimes for sheer survival. The hardships that Valerie, Marian and Alice faced seem unacceptable to some people and if she had been in that position Yvonne, as she says on p. 9. was sure she would have gone through with the termination that she called off at the last moment.

We have talked elsewhere in this book about the resilience and confidence you need when you have a baby and how, as a woman over 30, you may be able to make use of resources and expertise you have gained over the years. If you are a single parent, or become one at whatever stage after your child is born, those strengths are going to be even more vital. Marian's final word shows the conflicts very clearly:

> Only have a baby if you want it almost more than life itself. You need this strength of feeling to draw on when the baby will not stop crying and you come close to battering it at 3 a.m. or 4 a.m. or 5 a.m. or 6 a.m., any time from three weeks onwards. You *must* know that at bottom you really feel positive about this baby.
> The best things are everything about the baby. He is perfect! Happy, healthy, content, a good looking baby, good tempered,

very easy to handle. He casts joy about him – he is very popular with all babysitters, he is a terrific up-cheerer and brings a sort of magic with him. I could sit and watch him for hours – I feel so lucky to have such a darling – he's everything I could ever have wished for. I feel he's especially precious because I made myself wait for him (as I had to make sure of getting him).

10

Staying at Home: Being a Full-Time Mother

I had been teaching for 13 years when I became pregnant and decided to resign from my job as Head of English in a large comprehensive school. I was glad of the chance to do something else as I had become progressively disenchanted with the job. It was horrifying to think that I had spent 30 years in educational institutions without interruption.

Questioning the myths

However, as has been said in other chapters, there can be a difference between how you imagine it's going to be to stay at home with the baby and the reality. I was beguiled by romantic notions of the peaceful domestic life which was planned to be a welcomed contrast to those busy years of work – I was going to make bread and soup, learn to sew, conquer my hatred of gardening and do all the things the job had never allowed time for. Later, much later, I would find some part-time work. It didn't work out like that. Ben was a very alert and wakeful baby and there was little time to carry out my plans. Clearly it makes a big difference if you have a much more amenable baby like Aleid's:

> People keep asking me if I don't want to work – sometimes I feel it's a bit hard to feel that I *ought* to want to work. Twenty years ago it would have been quite abnormal if you did work but it is so much a thing that's done nowadays that I'm quite an exception.

Sometimes I think am I becoming uninteresting, have I got nothing to talk about? But in fact, in myself, I find it tremendously interesting. I really enjoy it. I really love doing things with my hands. It's so down to earth. I bought myself a sewing machine and I've started to sew which is lovely because I've never done that. I do lots of knitting and I paint and I enjoy it. I'm afraid that if I did go out to work it would all involve so much organizing.

For the first ten months of Ben's life I spent almost all of my time with him. Sometimes I felt very bored and frustrated which doesn't seem at all surprising now. The fact that I had happily anticipated spending all of every day with him, without realizing what that would be like, shows how strongly I had taken in and been taken in by the myth that all good mothers enjoy being with their small children all the time. Myths, which are often class-or culture-bound, also change frequently – the myth of romantic motherhood needs to change faster than some!

Practical considerations

Housework If you are looking after your child all day, you may also expect or be expected to look after the place where you live. For many women being a full-time mother also means being a full-time housewife. If you are over 30 and have been working, you will have developed a rhythm of fitting housework into your working life – your lives, if you live with other people. Having a baby and not going back to work may change that rhythm. It takes a perceptive partner to see that looking after a baby is not the same as looking after the home – they are not two sides of the same coin but two distinct jobs.

It may even be difficult to see that yourself and it is worth thinking this out at a very early stage. It is one of the greatest causes of later resentment between partners. Some women think that doing the housework would be a fair swap for being supported while you stay at home to care for the baby. The practical running of your lives will become your 'work'. But for many people that is not a satisfying job. It is hard work being with a baby all day. There are no bus journeys or coffee breaks to give space to unwind, especially if the baby is an unpredictable sleeper as many are. If you are looking after your child then that is your work, even if it is recognized only in terms of the derisory child benefit.

Nobody questions that looking after a baby is work when someone other than the mother does it – a nanny or a nursery nurse or a childminder is paid for looking after children, even if sometimes she is paid very little. If a mother decides to go back to work she will almost certainly have to pay someone else to do the work she was doing for free. To assume that a full-time mother will do all the housework as well, even if it means working until mid-evening and every weekend, is to confuse the issue quite dramatically. But it is a traditional trap that is very easy to fall into.

Housework is just as boring and repetitive as much factory or routine work but there is no wage packet at the end of the week. Because you have to decide what to eat, can't help noticing that the toothpaste has run out, and live amongst the unwashed dishes, it affects you much more than a routine job – you never get away from it but you still don't get paid. Housework is a necessary chore and it should be shared by the people who benefit from it. That isn't to say that it is not often possible to enjoy housework. Cooking can be creative and relaxing when you're in the mood and have time for it, and it can even be quite satisfying to restore order out of the chaos of toys and mess. When you're very busy and not too tired, the mindlessness of housework can be almost soothing. But if you're looking after a baby and housework is the only other thing you do, it is just that mindlessness that gets you down.

Money Giving up your job carries with it another very important implication: you give up the money you earned in that job. If you have been used to earning your own living or contributing your earnings to the running of the household, perhaps for 10–15 years, there is a good deal of adjusting to do when that money stops coming in.

When you were working you might well have taken on financial commitments that make a real difference now you're not. The change in the mortgage rate, for example, from 9 to 15 per cent within a very short space of time, made a nonsense of many people's economic planning. Janice:

> There have been great financial changes because I was working too. We've always had a joint account and shared our money so there was no difference there – it's just that there's much less of it and more to feed. I miss having money which I

know I earned because I feel guilty buying anything for myself
and so does Donald now that we have children. We keep
meaning to have a 'self-indulgence' fund but we haven't got
round to it yet. Of course, compared with many people we are
comfortably off and we have only just had to start budgeting
carefully as the economic restrictions have bitten into our
income. We try not to have to buy more than two pairs of
children's shoes in one month. We knew things would be
harder but the hardest thing was having to move house after
the birth of our fourth (not planned!) because we couldn't
afford to go on living where we were.

The drop in income may be marginally less dramatic for some
older parents when both of you have been earning for several
years. You may have savings and most of the equipment you
need and the feeling that you have contributed to that feeling of
security cushions the initial adjustment.

For some women being financially dependent on someone else
is worse than simply having less money. The resentment often
stems from the low public regard for the work of mothering –
seen as morally important and supposedly uplifting but of no
economic account. Diane:

> Dependency is a state of mind more than any actual reflection
> of who earns what. Certainly it is no reflection on my husband
> or his attitude to money. I still organize family finances, pay
> all bills, draw cash and usually decide what we can or cannot
> afford as I've always done. In fact I think it's more a question
> of self-image. I vehemently object to having to use the term
> 'housewife', partly because of the picture it creates of
> subservient little woman, and partly because I actually spend
> very little time doing housework, but then there's no satisfac-
> tory way of describing oneself in any other way. The term itself
> suggests economic dependency.

Being flexible One of the reasons you have a less organized day
with a small baby is because babies are extremely unpredictable.
Even if your baby seems to have established a reliable pattern,
you can be quite sure that the one time you really *want* her to go
to sleep/not to go to sleep/wake up/be happy to travel in the car
she'll do something different. That's Sod's Law. This is an area
that women over 30 find particularly difficult to deal with and it's
easy to see why. Years and years have been spent making

arrangements to fit all sorts of things into your life, adapting to the unexpected at times but feeling fairly certain of the parameters. Aleid describes how hard that is for her on p. 10 and Lesley found it similarly difficult (see p. 132).

It can take a long time to acknowledge that the skills and standards that made you good at your job, say, do you no good at all with a baby or a young child. You can no longer decide to do something and get it done as you used to do, because there is always another person whose needs and wishes are very different, saying 'What about me?'. I found this unquestionably the most difficult adjustment to make. Ben would happily tolerate my superficial attention being elsewhere as long as I could talk to him or let him help me – so cooking was usually OK, or washing up, or sweeping. But he wouldn't let me get a pen in my hand without saying 'mine!' or let me sort through a sheaf of papers without grabbing at them and even a glimpse of the typewriter sent him into a frenzied attempt to get at it. He wasn't stupid. The very things that used to be the tools of my trade – books, pens, papers, typewriter, not to mention uninterrupted conversation – were the things he wouldn't let me near. Quite right too, in his terms. He recognized the competition. The more I wanted to do something, the more it shut him out.

Isolation Much has been written about the isolation of women who spend most of their time at home. Since Betty Friedan's and Hannah Gavron's writings,[1] women are more aware of the dangers and yet it can still happen to you if you are unlucky or depressed or don't take real steps to see that it doesn't. The close one-to-one relationship that evolves out of a mother spending large chunks of time with a small baby can be difficult and feel unnatural. It is a very recent development and perhaps not a healthy one.

Much will depend on where you live and the sort of support network you already have. If your group of friends doesn't include people who are at home with their own babies, you will need to make contact with people who are around during the day. This was brought home very forcibly to Ray who looked after his son on his own for a week when Thomas was 15 months old:

Suddenly I was in somebody else's shoes . . . in the place of a mother really because Sally had gone away on holiday.

Although I enjoyed the week immensely, I did feel tremendously cut off and isolated and I was really glad that although I was on holiday, I had my own job in the back of my mind. I saw then how isolated it must be if that's all you do all day, look after children.

The social contacts Sally had built up had arisen out of her life with Thomas – they weren't part of her and Ray's life together and they were not connected with her job. Having a network of other women to see and spend time with is enormously important but it can lead to misunderstanding by some men who see those contacts not as a *necessary* support system but a frivolous, enjoyable way of spending your time while he is at work. David said:

> We almost had rows about the way her life had become much more middle class. A lot of time is taken up with groups. She had lots of people dropping in. During term-time I don't do anything really but work and there she is actually socializing although she's working at the same time, but it's a very different sort of work. Somehow living off the fat of the land while I'm working away.

That sort of socializing isn't always as attractive as it seems. You may not really enjoy sitting round chatting and having cups of tea as often as you end up doing it. You might rather be doing something more purposeful but it can be preferable to being alone at home with your baby if that is your only alternative.

Building up a support network Various suggestions are made on p. p. 134 about finding ways of getting some time on your own without your baby. That list is possibly more important to full-time mothers who don't get an organized break in the week, but it is placed there because it matters to all mothers. A number of the contacts you make who will give you some time away from your baby will also give you support at other times. There are other things you can do too to make life easier for you if you're at home with your baby.

Try and build up *local* contacts. You may have old friends who will mean a lot to you but if they are at work or live some distance away, you can't rely on them all the time. You need a few people who live within walking distance whom you can invite over for a cup of tea or drop in on for half an hour. Knowing that you can do that can sometimes give a focus to an otherwise unstructured day.

Find out from your health visitor or Well-Baby clinic or the library what groups there are in your neighbourhood – Mother and Baby, Meet-a-Mum and Mother and Toddler groups operate in church halls, community centres, attached to some play groups and in some primary schools. If you don't know many other women with children this may be something you will enjoy and it is a good opportunity to meet people. I made the mistake of thinking it wasn't appropriate to go to a Mother and Toddler group until you've got a toddler. Babies are fascinated by other children and your six-month-old baby might really enjoy watching someone else's toddler.

The NCT (National Childbirth Trust) has many groups all over the country that meet on a regular basis. These are usually organized in neighbourhoods, but even if you have to travel to one, it can be worth the effort as Tessa found:

> I made a lot of friends through my local NCT Postnatal Support Group in Harrogate. I found that I was given more help and encouragement from those mothers who had already 'been through it all', than from any other quarter.
>
> If I had not known about the group I think I would have felt very isolated and lonely as I have made no like-minded friends in the village where I live. I first went to the group when Charlotte was only three weeks old, and in the early weeks it was the focus of the whole week and meant a tremendous lot to me.

If you don't know of a local NCT group in your area, write to the head office and ask for your nearest group (see Address List on p. 213).

Perhaps you also went to an NCT antenatal class. If so, you should find that you are allocated a *postnatal supporter* – a woman who has at least one child and who knows what it's like. She will contact you after the birth and although you might not feel you want or need her help then, don't be reticent if you do need it later. Yvonne is a single parent:

> I did miss the chance for help when it was offered. The NCT had a postnatal supporter and she came and said, 'Hello, I'm

your contact. Here's my phone number if you need me.' And I never did ring. Never having done it, I felt a bit embarrassed about doing it two months later because I'd never established a relationship with her.

A neighbourhood *babysitting circle* can be an excellent support, not just in being able to use the babysitting facilities. There will probably be occasional meetings for parents and children to get to know each other and that will increase your local contacts.

You may feel that you want to meet people who have nothing to do with babies. This could be a *woman's group* in your area or a *class* run by the WEA (the Workers' Educational Association). Local education authorities (LEA) also run classes for adults in the daytime as well as evening classes. Some groups and classes have crèche facilities. Ask at your local library for information about what happens near you. To find out whether there are women's groups that might suit you, look in the local Women's Liberation newsletter if there is one, or write to WIRES which collects that sort of information on a national level (see Address List on p. 214).

Some women (and I confess I'm one of them) do not really enjoy coffee mornings or large gatherings of women and children. It may suit you better to set up much more *informal arrangements* on a fairly regular basis with fewer people involved. For example, I had a very fluid arrangement with three or four other women that on one afternoon a week, two of us would look after all the children. We took turns in each other's houses so it was quite varied. It meant that it wasn't such hard work or so boring with another adult to share the load and every three or four sessions you'd get one off. This was a sanity-saving scheme on Sunday afternoons one winter!

Swapping babies is an excellent way of getting yourself some free time to do something you want to do without it costing anything. This involves finding another woman with a child and arranging for one of you to look after both children at specified times so that the other is free. It is well worth starting this sort of scheme *early*, before the baby is five months if you can manage it. It may be harder work to have two small babies for a short time but if you leave it much longer, the baby is likely to be much more mother-dependent which makes it much harder to leave her. How often you do this or for how long will depend on you – some people do a half-day session, others manage a whole day, especially as the children get older. It helps to be able to leave a phone number in the early days while you're all getting used to the scheme. Another great help is to club together and buy a double buggy which you share, which means that you can always take the babies out. Living near the person you swap with obviously also makes a difference.

11

Working Mothers

If you are over 30 when you have your first child you may well be in a responsible and rewarding job which you don't want to give up. Alternatively, you may feel, as I did, that the job you hold would be incompatible with spending a fair amount of time looking after your baby yourself. However, simply because you are older you may have worked yourself into a position where you have more leverage about flexible working hours for example, or work that can be done at home.

Some professional jobs combine quite well with looking after a baby as long as they are not so demanding in themselves that there is little energy left over. This depends on the content of the job, how many hours 'full-time' means and how much work is taken home with you, literally or in your head. Teachers, nurses, doctors, university lecturers often manage to go back to their jobs although many mothers try to work part-time hours while their babies are small. Other women are already in freelance work which can continue. The greatest difficulties are experienced by women in executive positions that involve many unpredictable meetings or conferences or those in jobs (like television production or acting) that involve travelling or being away from home. For those women, unless they have a co-operative partner with very flexible working hours himself, a live-in nanny is the only possible way of continuing the job.

Although it is much more common for middle-class women to return to work after having a baby than it is for working-class women, there are still comparatively few women who return earlier than the 29 weeks' maternity leave and many of them return with a slightly different viewpoint. Current national figures show that only 6 per cent of women work full-time before their children are four years old.[1]

There has been a tremendous increase in the proportion of *mothers* who are in paid employment. By 1981 more than 50 per cent of women in Britain with children between the ages of five and nine went out to work but only 25 per cent of those with children under four.[2] This disparity is not because so many mothers of pre-school children *want* to stay at home with their children but because facilities for childcare are so inadequate that many of them have no choice. A fuller description of childcare options follows later in this chapter but underpinning the work aspirations of all mothers is the fact that childcare is placed very low indeed on the state's list of useful or necessary welfare provision. We are worse off for state childcare facilities in Britain than almost any country in Europe. And even once the children go to school, which is when many mothers try to return to work, school hours do not fit in with the full-time working day.

Any amount of talk and legislation about equal opportunities for women will not affect this huge disparity until society's view about bringing up children changes completely. Men and women ought to be able to bring up their children jointly, but to enable that to happen there would have to be more flexible working hours, a shorter working week, paternity as well as maternity leave and *much* better state-provided childcare facilities – a revolution indeed. However, given that there isn't enough work to go round and yet that some people (particularly men) have to spend so much time at work that they can spend very little time with their children, it would make sense to rethink work patterns in a radical way.

Doing two jobs

There is evidence that working mothers become less ambitious and are less likely to apply for promotion or take on extra responsibility. This, of course, has an enormous effect on the place of women in society. There are so few women in powerful jobs in any sphere of work, not because they are not able to do the jobs as competently as men, but because they always have two jobs to do.

Unless you have a lot of money and an unusually domesticated partner, you might well find yourself doing one job at work and another that starts as soon as you get home. This involves an enormous amount of organization, both practically in terms of your time and mentally, deciding on priorities. In her book *Double Identity: The Lives of Working Mothers*, Sue Sharpe says, 'It is ironic that the organization involved in combining home and childcare and a job would qualify many women for a management diploma, yet it goes unrecognized outside the home.'[3]

Fiona works as a lecturer in a College of Further Education. The way she describes how she and her partner organize their day shows that it is manageable but demanding. There is little room for anything to go wrong. Her daughter spends the day with a nursery nurse who also looks after two other children.

> When I'm at work I keep my mind on the job – I don't think about Caroline at all. I know she is in good hands, loved and well cared for and I can immerse myself in my work. The preparation and marking which teaching involves and which has to be done in the evening after I have put her to bed are more problematical. When I pick her up and come home in the evening, all my time and attention is for her.
>
> Nick feeds the cats and I feed Caroline. Then we share playing with her and prepare our dinner between us and Nick cooks it while I bath Caroline and put her to bed. Then we both eat, he washes up and I make bottles for the next day, and only then, at about 8.30 p.m., can I start to think about work. This is fine as long as I'm not going to be interrupted and can work as late as necessary. This has usually been so since she's started sleeping through the night at nine and a half weeks; but there have been periods when imminent teeth, nappy rash or a cold, or just a spell of colder weather, prevented her sleeping through the night and often her first waking would be before I went to bed, while I was still marking a pile of essays needed for 9 a.m. the next day, for example. This does quickly produce a feeling of strain.

Fiona's ability to cope with her job and her child depends fairly heavily, as she says, on other people – the nanny, her husband and, in an emergency, her neighbours. She also has to earn enough to be able to pay the nanny. From her account it sounds as if she has to have boundless energy, be pretty healthy and have a strong commitment to making it all work, which it clearly does, very well.

Working for 'pin-money'

There has been a very condescending view about the money married women earn when they go back to work. It is often assumed that the family does not *need* the money and that it is just an extra that will buy luxuries or pay for more interesting holidays. That assumption carries over into an assessment of the work women do as 'marginal' or 'secondary', at least not as important as the man's.[4] Even if a man is unemployed or earning less than a woman, she will rarely be seen as the breadwinner.

Although there are women over 30 who can afford a choice about not working, this is not so for everybody. Single women have a choice of working or living off the state. Couples where the man's earnings are very low or he is unemployed also have little choice about whether the woman should work. Some other couples, perhaps particularly older ones, commit themselves financially to a mortgage or dependants or emotionally to a style of life that makes it impossible to live off one income. Shirley shares a problem encountered by a number of first-time mothers in their thirties. Rising divorce rates often followed fairly quickly by remarriage means that there are now quite a lot of women having a first baby with a partner who already has children from a previous relationship:

> I was a principal teacher of guidance before I had the baby and after, as I returned when Beth was 29 weeks. My attitude to work/baby is an ongoing problem with me – unsolved as yet. I enjoy my job, but would prefer to be with the baby, but my husband's financial commitment from his previous marriage makes it impossible just now.

What you get out of working

All the way through this book we have seen women who say that their sense of self, their *self-esteem and confidence*, were connected with their work. This is generally recognized as a factor in the lives of all working mothers but perhaps it is more strongly felt by women who have been working for longer. Marcia works part-time as a vet after having her first child at 32: 'Although I didn't actually plan to be a working mum I'm now glad I managed to get established in my career before I had children. If I hadn't, I don't think I'd have had the confidence to take it up again.'

Studies of working mothers all seem to agree that having a job gives women much more than what they earn, especially if the alternative is to stay at home full-time with small children or be a 'housewife'. This is borne out by the contributors to this book: it seems that having more to do gives you more energy; the variety of activities that you do at work and at home compensates for the extra organization and tiredness; some jobs carry intrinsic rewards and satisfaction; there is an upsurging of confidence that you operate entirely separately in the 'real' world of work out there as well as being your baby's mother. In a study of women with pre-school children, Mary Boulton says, 'Few tasks are as harassing as caring for small children and the responsibility of other duties is compensated for by the respite from child care.'[5]

Another aspect of work that is very important and clearly makes the most tedious, unpleasant jobs tolerable is *the company* you get at work. Being at home with the baby can be isolating and lonely and going back to work can change all that. Julie went back to work part-time as a social worker when her baby was seven months old: 'It was very difficult for me to get a part-time job. I wanted to go back and I needed to for financial reasons but I didn't realize how lonely and isolated I'd feel at home. I think I couldn't have coped if I hadn't had my job, if I hadn't got away from him for a little while.' Julie's husband would have preferred her not to go back to work but he didn't put too much pressure on her. Some men who have a very traditional view of the role of a wife and mother object more strongly to their wives going out to work, especially if the extra money isn't vital. Many women resist these objections and work in spite of them but that can create tension. Linda was almost 40 when she had her first baby shortly after she was married:

> Before having a baby I was a personnel officer and I missed the people very much. I still do, after three years at home. I would have liked to return to it but this would not have been acceptable to my husband. I can't argue that I go without anything but I am very conscious of the fact that I don't earn any money, having been on a high salary with my own flat and car.

If your view of yourself changes when you have a baby, so does the way *other people* see you. On the one hand you have the comfortable sense of gaining approval by becoming a mother but, on the other hand, you might be treated as if you are quite a different person as a result. Jane had her first baby when she was 31 and working on a community magazine:

> I took the baby back with me to work when he was five weeks old. It was probably one of the most difficult times of my life. Lack of sleep, hard work and a feeling of guilt that I was not giving him enough attention.
>
> I was profoundly shocked by the social reactions to having a child. As a fairly attractive woman – childless – I could command a certain amount of respect and attention but after the birth I suddenly felt people stopped listening to what I said. Many emotional labels were put on me when I was basically doing the same job.
>
> I went to the central library to continue my research work for the magazine. I'd been there dozens of times before and I assumed that because I was breastfeeding there would be little problem. The baby rarely cried and if he did I simply put him to the breast to feed or to sleep. The librarian wouldn't let me come into the research room. She would not get me the articles I asked for. She was about 27 years old and simply refused to have the baby in the room. 'Come back without him,' she said. I asked a fellow researcher to sit in the canteen with him while I rushed through my work.

Reactions like that librarian's are extremely off-putting and disheartening especially since they often seem to come from other women who don't have children themselves. Another subtle sort of pressure can come from women who stayed at home with their children and then criticize you for working. Helena found this when she returned to her senior position in a modern languages' department at the school:

> One woman in the department who is in her forties put a lot of pressure on me. She'd say little things like 'It's so nice being at home with a child all day', or, 'It's so good for the children to have their mother around.' She knew all along that I felt strongly about it, that I wanted to come back. She resents now being at school and not being in the sort of position she might have been in if she'd stayed at work. I didn't find any pressure

from male members of staff but then when I came to the school
I made my views known and I was labelled a feminist!

Perhaps both of those reactions seems a bit like sour grapes but
you need to be feeling good for them not to get you down.

How important is the mother?

Most working mothers feel some guilt about working and some of
this arises from the current orthodoxy about mother–child
relationships and bonding first put forward by John Bowlby in
the 1950s. His ideas have led to some valuable changes in
institutions for young children and in obstetric practice, for
example, at the time of birth. However, as there have been more
and more working mothers since then, it has been possible to
research the effects of separation in more detail.

In the most substantial reassessment of maternal deprivation,
which looks at the evidence of a large number of studies of infant
and child behaviour, Michael Rutter says, 'Of course in most
families the mother has most to do with the young child and as a
consequence she is usually the person with whom the strongest
bond is formed. But it should be appreciated that the chief bond
need not be with the biological parent, it need not be with the
chief caretaker and it need not be with a female.'[6] In other words,
babies have fathers too – and grandmothers and uncles,
neighbours, childminders and siblings. Young children should be
able to make lasting bonds with a number of people, not
necessarily all adults, and the implied suggestion is that it may
actually be harmful for a young child, especially the first child, to
spend all her time exclusively with her mother in the isolated way
that is now relatively common even though very new.

All of this needs to be said much more loudly and clearly if
mothers are to feel less guilty when they leave their children. We
need to hear from people like Heather who, because she is a
single parent, had to go back to work:

> I have to be honest – I don't worry about him at all. It was a
> fantastic relief. I felt I was an amateur mother. I didn't really
> know what I was doing and that the childminder who was
> used to looking after children would be able to look after him
> ten times better than I could. Somebody with experience,
> other kids around – it was an enormous relief. It can still be a
> blessed relief to go to work on a Monday morning.

The evidence does seem to suggest that a child's separation from her mother while the mother is working does not have a detrimental effect as long as the quality of the childcare is good. Given that, there may actually be an advantage in the intensity and the *quality of the time* you spend with your child when you are not working. You're both pleased to see each other; you haven't had time to get on each other's nerves or be bored; weekends take on a new enjoyment.

Research carried out by Rhona and Robert Rapaport on the work and lives of 1,000 male and female graduates looked closely at 16 dual-career families.[7] Several advantages were perceived for their children. Because of their busy lives, activities including the children tended to be planned more carefully and the parents developed close relationships with their children by their involvement when they were together. The children quickly accepted the importance of both parents' work and became more independent and resourceful if they were seen as necessary helpers in making things run smoothly. This seems to give weight to the idea that it is not the amount of time that you spend with your child that matters but what you do with the time you do spend together.

Alternatives to full-time work away from home

Part-time work This fits in much better with looking after a small child so it is easy to see why it is so attractive to mothers, enabling them to do their two jobs in fewer hours. However, part-time work in this country tends to be extremely badly paid compared with full-time work and you also lose most of your legal rights to sickness and unemployment benefit and maternity leave unless you fulfil certain stringent (and often impossible) conditions. Having to pay for childcare while you work part-time can mean that you can have very little money left over at the end of the week. If the job is interesting it is also possible to find yourself working extra hours for no pay at all.

Sue had had no doubt at all that she would go back to work full-time (as an infant teacher) before she had William: 'Then as soon as I had him I knew I wasn't going to do it. It was a big cloud on my horizon the day I had to go back. I didn't want to do it and it obsessed me for six months. I felt so responsible. Part-time work seemed a really happy medium. I wouldn't have been happy to be at home.' She was lucky enough to get a part-time teaching job, in itself a rarity, but not all jobs lend themselves to part-time hours.

Freelance work This may work out better if you are already familiar with it and have built up the necessary contacts. If you are over 30 this is more likely to be so. The flexibility of being able to work at or from home is a great advantage. Judy found things quite difficult when Justin was born but developing a way of continuing her work as a potter helped considerably.

> When Justin was two months old I hired a nanny to look after him three afternoons a week while I went to my studio and tried to work. It was very difficult to reacquire the discipline but I was now sure of an uninterrupted time in which to work. I had tried to work before but Justin was a very wakeful baby and was not content to lie quietly on his back while I tried desperately to finish my latest order, always weeks overdue. The constant interruption used to drive me insane.

It can be easier, if you work freelance, to arrange fixed times when someone else will look after your child. Even if you have the flexibility to take the baby with you, having to perform both roles simultaneously is very exhausting and you might feel better if you can concentrate on one at a time.

Working from home This involves a considerable amount of discipline but being over 30 probably helps you. Anna:

> You do have to be very strong with yourself, though, if you're to use the time you do get to yourself to do some real 'work'. You can always justify getting on with the cooking or housework, reading the newspaper, weeding the garden, catching up on sleep. But I'm sure it's easier to overcome these temptations if you have had a job and have laid down habits of work. My last job required a lot of self-discipline and self-motivation, and I feel that I'm drawing on that experience now.

If you do work at home and have little organized childcare, as I did when I started working on this book, you have to evolve methods of working that may be very different from your previous style. Yvonne was on secondment from her job when Sam was born and was taking an advanced diploma.

I remember reading somebody's analogy that a baby takes a day and throws it against the wall and smashes it into such small fragments that you can't piece them together. I had to learn to use my time differently. With my academic work I'd been used to clearing the decks and settling down for four or five hours. I had to learn to do it in 20-minute bursts, which was good.

Job-sharing In a few couples the man stays at home to look after the baby while the mother works, but that is still quite rare. A more equal way of sharing the childcare is also to share the job. This is also unusual but some people have been able to reorganize their working lives in a very interesting way. In some cases both partners have different part-time jobs, sometimes shared with someone else, e.g. two women share one job in a housing association. It is still very difficult to find employers prepared to consider such an arrangement in spite of the obvious advantages. Employers get the energy and expertise of two people rather than one. It is likely that this sort of arrangement works well for people in their thirties or forties who have already proved their competence in work and may have more resources to draw on. If you are interested in job-sharing, it is worth researching the possibilities very carefully. There is an organization that can help you, *New Ways To Work* (for the address, see p. 213).

It is often best to find the person yourself who could share the job so that you can work out proposed details in advance and apply for the job together. Some employers are flexible enough to consider a joint application for a job if you present your case very carefully, but it is probably better to approach it that way round rather than to ask first whether they would consider a job share.

Liz and Peter share the same job. Lucy was born when Liz was 36 and Peter 51.

Liz: Nominally I'm the job holder but it's up to me to delegate whatever I like. I'm coordinator of a Victims Support Scheme and that means contacting the police for any cases of victims of crime and then allocating them to volunteers to go and visit. There's a lot of back-up work. For one week I will do the telephoning, which is a morning's work, and Peter will be looking after Lucy. We change at lunchtime.
Peter: The job is home-based so that's the great thing about it. It just happens that there isn't much money in this particular

charity. We knew it was insecure when we took it on. We only got a year's contract and there's no pension scheme but we reckoned that to do something that fitted in with what we wanted to do with Lucy and to do something that was worth doing in itself was more important than a good salary and the usual fringe benefits that you expect from work.

Liz: Before we started I'd found it quite difficult to get used to being on my own at home (that lasted ten months). I think if you go on like that you end up by having quite different perceptions of the world. Particularly husbands who work in industry and don't come home till 6 p.m. When Peter was working full-time I used to envy my friends with teacher husbands who would be home just after 4 p.m. I'd think gosh, two hours to go. He'd come home and I'd say, 'Of course you don't know what it's been like,' if I had had a bad day and Pete would say, 'Well you don't know what it's been like stuck in a place without fresh air all day,' and you just acquire parallel tracks with hardly any time to meet, particularly if you tend to be busy in the evening with various things. That struck us particularly afterwards when we started seeing more of each other and having breakfast together and other civilized things.

Liz and Peter took what some people would see as a brave decision. Being older helped them to take that financial risk because they had had a chance to equip a household and save some money so they could then decide where their priorities lay.

More recently Liz wrote:

Lucy has just started school and I am thinking 'What next?' as I feel four and a half years in the present job is enough. So I'm aiming to move on soon, though I shall miss the job-sharing. From Lucy's point of view, the job-sharing has worked out really well – she has a good relationship with us both and expects 'basic care' from either of us (though she knows Peter is more likely to cook nice meals and I'm more likely to mend ripped clothes).

To a large extent Liz and Peter had to depend on their savings to enable them to carry out their job-sharing.

Cathy and John share the care of Claire and each works part-time. Financially it is difficult too: 'The deal has to be that if we share childcare then we both earn our own living and you're faced with trying to earn a living in two and half days a week.

From my point of view, the sharing is very much better than looking after her all the time but I wouldn't want to idealize it.'

Breastfeeding and work

One of the worries you may have if you want to return to work is whether you will be able to continue breastfeeding. It is perfectly possible to do this although it will be more difficult the younger the baby is. If your baby is exclusively breastfed you will need either to express enough milk for your absence or to get back to her to feed her, if you work near enough home. Alison continued feeding by having her baby brought to her office at work.

If you are going to rely on your own milk, you need to get used to expressing milk early so that it becomes easy for you and not another strain to cope with when you go back to work. Expressed milk will keep in the fridge for 24 hours and also freezes well. It is worth finding the kind of breast pump that will suit you best and take the least time. You will also need to get your baby used to accepting milk from a bottle. If you leave it too late (i.e. after she is more than a couple of months old) she may decide it is a poor substitute for your breast. Fiona:

> Knowing that she would have to have two bottles a day with her nanny once term started, I began at three months to try to introduce one bottle a day to get her used to it. How she hated it! My milk supply was now plentiful (with the help of a pint of Guinness a day) and it seemed a real shame to have to deny it to her, so we both got very upset over this wretched bottle and I would then give in to her furious screams and give her the breast. We then discovered a different kind of bottle with a teat shaped more like a human nipple and a system of pre-sterilized disposable plastic bottles and she took to it immediately. From three and a half months, therefore, she had two bottles and three breastfeeds, or if I was late picking her up, three bottles and two breast feeds. The supply of breast milk was kept up and she now (at eight months) has three solid meals a day with drinks of milk from a sucker cup and a breastfeed morning and evening. She does so enjoy her breastfeed and I must admit so do I, and I am very pleased that I am still able to give it.

If you are taking the 29 weeks' maternity leave there should be no problem about breastfeeding because by then you will probably only be feeding her morning and night anyway. If you are out at work, breastfeeding before you go and when you come back is a lovely way of spending close time together. The *La Lèche* League publishes further advice on combining breastfeeding and work (see p. 218).

Childcare

Most mothers who work have to make arrangements for someone else to look after their children. There are various possible forms this can take, which are briefly outlined below. The facilities provided in Britain by the state are extremely limited and becoming more so as the cuts bite. Voluntary organizations like the pre-school playgroups usually exist more with the needs of the child in mind than the working mother. Childcare facilities vary greatly from area to area so you would need to look carefully at your local provision.

Local Authority day nurseries These look after pre-school children for a full working day but there are massive waiting lists for places. The Local Authority targets for day care places is 8 per 1,000 children under five and full-time day care is only available for 0.7 per cent of all pre-school children.[8] Organized by the DHSS, these nurseries provide only for those who meet the definition of priority children and not all of them. If you are a single mother you might have a chance of a place in a day nursery, otherwise it is extremely unlikely. Day nurseries are staffed by NNEB-trained nursery nurses whose job is seen as caring for the children rather than educating them.

Nursery schools and classes There are provided by the DES for some of the children between three and five but only during school hours and terms which may well not suit a working mother. They are staffed by trained teachers often with a nursery nurse as an auxiliary helper. Here the emphasis is on pre-school education and it may be offered on a part-time basis, i.e. mornings or afternoons only. In certain areas there are waiting lists for nursery places so it is worth putting your child's name on the list early, by the time she is a year old. A small number of authorities also provide 'extended day nursery schooling' which enables the parent to work full-time hours but these are few and far between.

Play groups These are run by voluntary and community organizations and provide a large proportion of pre-school care after the age of three. Although they fulfil a real need and are very popular for the facilities they provide, they are not a reliable form of childcare for working mothers. They are usually open for only two to three hours and not always every day of the week. Many of them also involve mothers so you could not then also be free to work. There are a few play groups that operate an extended day to cater for the needs of working parents but they are very rare.

Childminders A great deal of pre-school childcare is undertaken by childminders, registered or not. Officially, childminders should be registered with the Local Authority but many mothers make their own arrangements for childminding with relatives, friends or neighbours. Because a childminder usually looks after the children in her own home, the hours can normally fit in with those of a working parent and it is by far the most popular system of childcare, particularly for babies and toddlers. Childminders are not trained, although there are now courses they can attend, and they fix their own hourly rates, most of which are much less than other private facilities. A childminder will often look after two or three children and possibly one of her own too.

Paula went back to work after four and a half months and shortly after that, her difficult relationship with her partner broke down. She felt very lucky in her childcare:

> I'm sure I only managed so well because I have such an excellent childminder. She is a lovely person with three children of her own, aged from 9 to 12. She is genuinely fond of children and seems quite devoted to the three she looks after, playing with them endlessly. The only snag is that she lives quite a long way away – it takes me about half an hour's walk – I don't have a car and the bus service is very poor. At the end of a working day, with heavy shopping to carry, it can seem like a long walk. However, I consider myself extremely fortunate to have someone so loving and so reliable. I pay her 18 pounds [this was 1981] and would pay more if I could afford it. Being a single mum is not an easy life but the tremendous joy and feeling of achievement that's derived from having a little baby around far outweigh the problems. I often think to myself 'this is the happiest I'll ever be'.

If you work full-time, a childminder is still expensive, though not as expensive as some other kinds of care. Heather, also a single parent, made her decision about when to go back to work on the basis of the cost to her of paying a childminder – she put it off as long as she could:

> I came back at the point that half-pay started – 14 weeks. I was so exhausted when I was at home I can remember thinking, I'm not going to be able to cope at work. My sister said, you mustn't worry about this. It is such a relief when someone else is looking after the baby that you'll find you have more energy than you deemed was possible. And she was *right*. I went back to work after dropping Tom off at the new childminder and I felt so much better straight away. I wished I'd gone back sooner.

Workplace nurseries There are a few workplace nurseries run by factories, companies, hospitals, universities and other institutions, but all together these provide a very small number of the total places for pre-school children. Those that operate in universities and colleges of higher and further education usually close during the vacations. Women who use a workplace nursery can, however, feel tied to their employer and, therefore, their job because they feel dependent on these facilities.

Private nurseries These have to be registered with the Social Services Department. They vary greatly in the facilities offered – training of staff, opening hours, the ages of the children they take and what they provide for them. Prices vary too but a full-time place in a private nursery staffed by trained people is likely to cost at least £30–35 a week. For reasons of cost alone, they will never meet the needs of many working mothers.

Sharing a nursery nurse An alternative to a private nursery in a separate building is offered by some nursery nurses. A trained nursery nurse or nanny will care for two, three or four children, basing herself in one of their homes, often on a rotating basis. Her salary is made up by the contributions of the different parents. This differs from childminding which is usually based in the home of the childminder herself. This is a popular form of childcare for working mothers but it is also expensive. Helena shares a nanny with one other parent and it costs them £120 each a month plus food for the nanny and both children during the fortnight they spend in her house each month. 'It's like taking out a second mortgage,' she says.

A nanny Having your own nanny come to your house to look after your child is probably the most convenient arrangement but undoubtedly the most expensive and therefore only open to the most highly paid. If she comes on a daily basis it will cost at least £35–40 a week. Yvonne, who lives alone now, has that sort of arrangement and although it costs her £150 a month, she prefers it to her previous choice – of offering a room in her house to an unmarried mother in return for childcare. 'It costs me more in cash terms that it did having Jenny living here but for that £150 a month I also get my privacy and solitude and have things my way. If I didn't pay £150 a month I couldn't go out and earn more than £150 a month. I think it's well worth it – I don't begrudge a penny of it.'

A live-in trained nanny is even more expensive. She will require £50–75 a week plus her own room, a television, her meals and her insurance contributions paid. A live-in mother's help (the name for someone who looks after your child but is *not* trained) will cost £35–40 a week plus her food. A nanny will expect to look after the child and her clothes and food but not to do other housework for you.

An au pair An au pair is someone (usually a teenage girl) from another country who lives in your house and does about 15 hours of childcare or light housework a week in return for a room, her food and about £15–£20 pocket money. She will usually be quite young, 18–20, will be here because she wants to learn the language rather than necessarily look after children, and will need some support in being treated as part of your family. She may not speak English well or be particularly interested in children so if you want an au pair to look after a small child you need to choose her very carefully.

Ad hoc arrangements Many working mothers have less formal arrangements for childcare, especially once the children go to school. A combination of grandmothers and other relatives, friends, neighbours, teenage girls at school, is used to take children to school and collect them and sometimes fill in the after-school hours until at least one parent is home. A surprising number of working mothers rely on these very informal arrangements.

Margaret took her first child to work with her for some time.

> I worked as a researcher in a School of Librarianship from 1970–9. After Harriet was born I worked part-time; I was amazingly lucky with childcare. At first she came with me in the carry-cot (anyway I was breastfeeding her all the time) and I gradually left her with the receptionist downstairs who got more involved and in the end Harriet just stayed down there all morning while I worked upstairs. Jane looked after her beautifully and could do her own work too and Harriet loved her and loved being there. It was super. But when my research project ended and I was expecting Robert it all came to an end.

What there should be It is fairly obvious from this overview how inadequate childcare facilities are. The Equal Opportunities Commission recommends that day care provision should be made available for all parents wanting to work or study. This provision should be available throughout the year, be close to the home or work- or study-place and have hours flexible enough to provide both full- and part-time care. It should also be available at a price parents can realistically afford. It should have staff sympathetic to the needs and circumstances of working/studying parents and standards of care should be adequate, both in the interests of the children and so that parents are free from anxiety when they leave their children. Facilities developed jointly by employers, unions and local authorities would achieve these aims much more successfully than the present compartmentalized system.

The campaign for better childcare facilities is hampered by the fact that the people who need it most – mothers with children – are either too busy or too tied to devote their energies to it. Even if they do, the period when their need is greatest will pass relatively soon and the campaign can lose impetus and continuity. To achieve a better system there needs to be a radical change of approach. Here is Sue Sharpe:

> We have to change the underlying attitudes towards substitute childcare, the very term denoting something inferior. While care outside the home is always assumed to be second best to

that within it, and while we try to reproduce the conditions of mothering in the family rather than extending relationships of love, trust and stability into other caring environments with other children and adults, we are denying potentially enriching experiences to all those concerned. There is no logical reason why childcare arrangements that best fulfil the interests of children, and those that satisfy the interests of their parents, should be in conflict.[9]

Rights of employment

The Employment Acts of 1975 and 1980 established certain minimal rights for working women who become pregnant as long as they fulfil certain conditions. However, proposals under consideration at the time of going to press threaten some of these rights. You should check whether the information that follows has changed. All women have the right to be paid for the time they take off work for antenatal care visits. Legally, an employer can ask to see a doctor's certificate.

Pregnancy and unfair dismissal If you are sacked from your job when you become pregnant or for any reason connected with your pregnancy, you must have been employed there for at least two years to claim unfair dismissal. If you can no longer do your job adequately 'because of your pregnancy' (because, say, you have to lift heavy weights) or if you work in a job where it is illegal or dangerous for the job to be done by a pregnant woman (e.g. radiology), you may be dismissed but you have the right to reinstatement 29 weeks after the birth. If either of these two positions apply to you, the employer should offer you an alternative job if there is one available before dismissing you. If you think you have been unfairly dismissed, you can complain to an Industrial Tribunal. However, the 1980 Employment Act has made it much more difficult to win a claim of unfair dismissal by making it easier for employers to justify the sacking.

Maternity leave If you have been working for the same employer for at least two years, and for at least 16 hours a week, you are entitled to six weeks' paid maternity leave at 90 per cent of your basic pay (see chapter 3, p. 66). You are also entitled to return to your job 29 weeks after the baby's birth.

To claim this entitlement you must remain in your job until

the eleventh week before your baby is due. *This is important*. You must also tell your employer that you intend to return to work. This must be done on two occasions and in writing: at least 21 days before you leave work and at least 21 days before the date you would like to start work again. Your employer may write to you while you are on maternity leave asking whether you intend to return to work and if this happens you must reply in writing within 14 days. Maternity pay is based on the last week's work before going on maternity leave, so don't start working part-time before that.

The right to your own job The 1980 Employment Act introduced changes that mean you may not necessarily get your original job back. Suitable alternative work must be offered if your own job is not available and it must be on terms and conditions 'not substantially less favourable' than your original job. But if you refuse this offer 'unreasonably', you completely lose your right to reinstatement. The job that is offered to you must be the same job as defined in your contract of employment so you need to check the exact wording of your contract to see what this means. It could mean that a teacher, for example, is offered a teaching job in a different school.

Continuity of employment The period of your maternity leave does affect the continuity of employment in terms of pension schemes and promotion prospects. This may be particularly important for older first-time mothers returning to work, because in some organizations there are age limits to certain kinds of promotion, which could mean the opportunity is lost.

Paternity leave Unlike many European countries, there is no officially recognized paternity leave in this country. Some unions have negotiated a week or more of paternity leave at the time of the birth but most men still have to take any time off as part of their holiday.

References

1 Choices and Decisions: Thinking Ahead

1 OPCS, *Birth Statistics* (HMSO, 1982) Series FM No. 9, p. 9.
2 OPCS, *Birth Statistics* (1982) Series FM No. 9, p. 11.
3 Joan Michelson and Sue Gee, *Coming Late to Motherhood* (Thorsons, 1984), p. 251.

2 Controlling your Fertility: Contraception and Conception

1 'Fertility in Older Women', *International Planned Parenthood Federation Medical Bulletin* 18 (2) (April 1984), 4–6.
2 AFFPA Medical Task Force, 'Guidelines on Contraception', *British Journal of Sexual Medicine* (October 1983), 33.

3 Pregnancy

1 Gordon Bourne, *Pregnancy* (Pan, 1975), p. 339.
2 N. R. Butler and E. Alberman, *Perinatal Problems* (Livingstone, 1969).
3 C. R. Stark, M. Orleans, A. D. Haverhamp and J. Murphy, 'Short and long-term risks after exposure to diagnostic ultrasound *in utero*', *Obstetrics & Gynaecology* 63 (1984), 194–200.
4 Royal College of Obstetricians and Gynaecologists, *Report of the ROCG working party on routine ultrasound examinations in pregnancy* (December 1984).

5 'An assessment of the hazards of amniocentesis', Report to the Medical Research Council by their working party on amniocentesis, *British Journal of Obstetrics and Gynaecology* 85 (1978), supplement 2, 1–41.
6 J. Philip and J. Bang, *British Medical Journal* 2 (1978), 1183–4.

4 The Birth

1 Sheila Kitzinger (ed.), *Episiotomy – Physical and Emotional Aspects* (National Childbirth Trust, 1981).
2 Katherina Dalton, *Depression after Childbirth: How to Recognize and Treat Postnatal Illness* (Oxford University Press, 1980).
3 Ann Oakley, 'Confinement and Depression', *Medicine in Society* 7 (1) (Spring 1981), 19–20.

5 The Risk to the Baby

1 Social Services Committee, House of Commons 1979–80, *Perinatal and Neonatal Mortality* (HMSO, 1980), commonly known as the Short Report.
2 Butler and Alberman, *Perinatal Problems*.
3 G. Chamberlain et al., *British Births 1970* (Heinemann, 1975) vol. 2, table 2.15.
4 D. Nortman, 'Parental age as a factor in pregnancy outcome and child development', *Reports on Population/Family Planning* 16, (1974), 1–52.
5 The Short Report, *Perinatal and Neonatal Mortality*, pp. 109–10.
6 P. M. Dunn, *The influence of the intrauterine environment in the causation of congenital postural deformities with special reference to congenital dislocation of the hip* MD thesis (University of Cambridge, 1969).
7 P. M. Dunn, 'Congenital Postural Deformities', *British Medical Bulletin* 32 (1) (1976), 71–6.
8 John O. Forfar and G. C. Arneil, *Textbook of Paediatrics* (Livingstone, 1979), p. 201.
9 Margaret and Arthur Wynn, *The Prevention of Handicap and the Health of Women* (Routledge & Kegan Paul, 1979), p. 12.
10 Butler and Alberman, *Perinatal Problems*, p. 51.
11 J. Fedrick and A. Anderson, *British Journal of Obstetrics and Gynaecology* 83 (May 1976), 342–50.

6 The First Six Weeks or So

1 Jill Tweedie, *The Guardian*, 2 February 1981.
2 Dana Breen, *The Birth of a First Child* (Tavistock Publications, 1975), pp. 90–1.
3 Jo Douglas and Naomi Richman, *My Child Won't Sleep* (Penguin, 1984), p. 20.

7 How You Feel About Yourself

1 Penelope Leach, *Baby and Child* (Penguin, 1977).
2 Douglas and Richman, *My Child Won't Sleep.*

8 You and Your Partner

1 Brian Jackson, *Fatherhood* (Allen & Unwin, 1983), p. 9 .
2 Michelson and Gee, *Coming Late to Motherhood*, p. 258.
3 Reported in *The Sunday Times*, 3 October 1982.
4 Michelson and Gee, *Coming Late to Motherhood*, pp. 256–7.

9 On Your Own: Being a Single Parent

1 Rita Craft, 'One in a Million', *The Chartist* 90 (April/May 1982).
2 Michelson and Gee, *Coming Late to Motherhood*, pp. 267–8.
3 Ibid., p. 269.

10 Staying at Home: Being a Full-Time Mother

1 Betty Friedan, *The Feminine Mystique* (Gollancz, 1963); Hannah Gavron, *The Captive Wife* (Routledge & Kegan Paul, 1966).

11 Working Mothers

1 OPCS, *General Household Survey* (HMSO, 1981), table 4.14.
2 OPCS, *General Household Survey* (1981), table 4.15.
3 Sue Sharpe, *Double Identity: the Lives of Working Mothers* (Penguin, 1984), p. 233.
4 These terms are used as defined by Pauline Hunt in *Gender and Class Consciousness* (Macmillan, 1980).
5 Mary G. Boulton, *On Being a Mother* (Tavistock Publications, 1983), p. 195.
6 Michael Rutter, *Maternal Deprivation Re-assessed* (Penguin, 1981), p. 127.
7 Rhona and Robert Rapaport, *Dual Career Families* (Penguin, 1971).
8 Equal Opportunities Commission, '*I want to work . . . but what about the kids*? (EOC, 1978).
9 Sue Sharpe, *Double Identity*, p. 134.

Useful Addresses

Association for Breastfeeding Mothers (ABM), 131 Mayow Road, London SE26. 24-hour counselling service (01–461 0022).

Association for Improvement in Maternity Services (AIMS), 163 Liverpool Road, London N1 0RF (01–278 5628).

Association for Postnatal Illness, 7 Gowan Avenue, Fulham, London SW6. Send SAE for information and advice.

Association for Smoking and Health (ASH), 27 Mortimer Street, London W11.

British Acupuncture Association, 34 Alderney Street, London SW1. Send SAE and £1.50 for list of qualified practitioners and information.

British Homeopathic Association, 27a Devonshire Street, London W1N 1LJ. Send SAE and £1.00 for list of registered practitioners.

British Pregnancy Advisory Service, 2nd Floor, 58 Petty France, Victoria, London SW1 (01–222 0985). Referral service with information about clinics in other cities.

Centre of Advice on Natural Alternatives (CANA), Tyddyn y Myndydd, Llanelly Hill, Gwent (0873–831182). Send SAE for information.

Compassionate Friends, c/o Gill Hodder, 5 Lower Clifton Hill, Bristol BS8 1BT (0272–292778). Support group for bereaved parents.

Cry-Sis, 63 Putney Road, Enfield, Middlesex EN3 6NN (01–822 4720). Support for parents whose babies cry excessively.

DAWN, St Clement's DDA, 2a Bow Road, London E3. Help for women with drink problems.

Down's Children's Association, 4 Oxford Street, London W1 (01–580 0511/2).

Feminist Library and Information Centre, Hungerford House, Victoria Embankment, London WC2N 6PA (01–930 0715).

Foresight, Association for the promotion of preconceptual care, c/o Mrs P Barnes, Woodhurst, Hydestile, Godalming, Surrey GU8 4AY (048 68–5743).

Gingerbread, 35 Wellington Street, London WC2 (01–240 0953).

Hyperactive Children's Support Group (HACGS), c/o Sally Bunday, 59 Meadowside, Angmering, West Sussex BN16 4BW (0243–551313).

The Lady, 40 Bedford Street, London WC2. Carries advertisements for nannies.

La Lèche League, BM 3424, London WC1V 6XX (01–404 5011). Information and advice on breastfeeding.

Meet-a-Mum Association (MAMA), National Organizer: Mary Whitlock, 26a Cumnor Hill, Oxford OX2 9HA. Local groups put mothers in touch with each other.

National Association for the Welfare of Children in Hospital (NAWCH), Argyle House, 29–31 Euston Road, London NW1 2SD (01–261 1738).

National Childbirth Trust (NCT), 9 Queensborough Terrace, London W2 3TB (01–221 3833). Also local branches.

National Childcare Campaign, c/o Surrey Docks Childcare Project, Docklands Settlement, Redriff Road, London SE16.

National Childminders' Association, 13 London Road, Bromley, Kent BR1 1DE.

The National Children's Centre, Longroyd Bridge, Huddersfield, West Yorkshire (0484–41733). Register of parents' help-lines; 24-hour answerphone.

National Council for One Parent Families, 255 Kentish Town Road, London NW5 2LX (01–267 1361).

Natural Family Planning Centre, c/o Mrs S Burton, Birmingham Maternity Hospital, Birmingham B15 2TG (021–472 1377 ext. 102).

National Housewives Register (NHR), 245 Warwick Road, Solihull, West Midlands B92 7AH (021–706 1101). Also local groups.

New Ways to Work, 347a Upper Street, London N1 (01–226 4026). Information about jobsharing.

Organization for Parents Under Stress (OPUS), 26 Manor Drive, Pickering, North Yorkshire YO18 8DD.

Pre-Eclamptic Toxaemia Society (PETS), c/o Dawn James, 88 Plumberrow, Lee Chapel North, Basildon, Essex SS15 5LP. A self-help group for women with high blood pressure in pregnancy.

Society to Support Home Confinement, c/o Margaret Whyte, 17 Laburnham Avenue, Durham City (0385–61325).

Stillbirth and Neonatal Death Society (SANDS), 37 Christchurch Hill, London NW3 1LA (01–794 4601).

Wires, National Women's Liberation Newsletter and Information Service, PO Box 20, The Centre, Oxford (0865–240991).

Useful Books

Pregnancy and Childbirth

New Life: A Book of Exercises for Pregnancy and Childbirth, Janet and Arthur Balaskas (Sidgwick & Jackson, 1983). Yoga-based exercises to achieve maximum flexibility in childbirth. Good photographs and helpful drawings.

The Childbirth Book, Christine Beels (Turnstone Books, 1978). A feminist approach to giving birth which helps women to retain control of their own bodies during childbearing. Contains details of co-operation card.

Pregnancy, Gordon Bourne (Pan, 1975). A detailed account of pregnancy and childbirth by a consultant obstetrician with a traditional approach.

The Pregnancy After 30 Workbook, Ed. Gail Sforza Brewer (Rodale Press, USA, 1978). An American book not easily available here. Worth seeking out for its positive and reassuring information and advice.

Sooner or Later: The Timing of Parenthood in Adult Lives, Pamela Daniels and Kathy Weingarten (W. W. Norton, 1982). An interesting and very detailed American study that covers any risks very thoroughly. Based on research supported by the Wellesley College Center for Research on Women.

The New Good Birth Guide, Sheila Kitzinger (Penguin, 1983). Lists detailed information about maternity hospitals. Helpful in choosing where to give birth.

Pregnancy and Childbirth, Sheila Kitzinger (Michael Joseph, 1980).
A comprehensive guide to pregnancy, labour and early
parenthood. Sensible, reassuring approach which pays attention to feelings too. Contains details of co-operation card.

You might like to read other books by Sheila Kitzinger – she
has written many! *The Experience of Childbirth* (Penguin, 1970);
The Experience of Breastfeeding (Penguin, 1979) and *Birth Over
Thirty* (Sheldon Press, 1982).

Your Baby, Your Body, Your Life, Angela Phillips (Allen & Unwin,
1984). Lively, cheering guide to pregnancy and birth. Very
positive and helpful and clearly written from recent experience.

Self-Insemination, A pamphlet available from Sisterwrite, 190
Upper Street, London N1. Gives advice and information about
how to go about it.

Motherhood

With Child: A Diary of Motherhood, Phyllis Chesler (Thomas Y.
Crowell, New York, 1979). A beautifully written personal
journal by an American feminist. Particularly revealing about
her difficulties of trying to live and work as a mother.

Rocking the Cradle: A Challenge in Family Lives, Ed. Gillian E
Hanscombe and Jackie Forster (Peter Owen, 1981). An
account of the perspective of lesbian mothers based on
interviews with them – raises important issues about being a
mother and a lesbian.

Coming Late to Motherhood, Joan Michelson and Sue Gee (Thorsons, 1984). The personal stories of twenty women who had
their first babies over thirty – a compulsive read.

From Here to Maternity, Ann Oakley (Penguin, 1981). Interviews
form the basis for this interesting study of various aspects of
motherhood.

Of Woman Born, Adrienne Rich (Virago, 1977). A theoretical
exploration of the personal, psychological and political issues
of motherhood, based on her experiences, by a well-known
American feminist poet.

Postnatal Depression, Vivienne Welburn (Fontana, 1980). A
helpful book that draws on personal experience and offers
support.

Childrearing

Coping Alone, Clara Clark (The Women's Press, 1982). A mixture of advice, information and personal experience about being a single parent.

What To Do When There's Nothing To Do, Boston Children's Medical Center and Elizabeth M Gregg (Arrow Books, 1984). Practical suggestions for staving off boredom with small children.

Living With a Toddler, Brenda Crowe (Allen & Unwin, 1982). Acknowledges that toddlers can be hard work and has all sorts of suggestions for dealing with them.

My Child Won't Sleep, Jo Douglas and Naomi Richman (Penguin, 1984). Particularly helpful for suggesting ways of dealing with irregular sleep patterns in babies and young children.

Baby and Child, Penelope Leach (Penguin, 1979). A detailed, comprehensive, useful manual about the first five years. Lots of helpful advice and practical suggestions, seen from the baby's point of view.

All About Twins: A Handbook for Parents, Gillian Leigh (Routledge & Kegan Paul, 1983). Information and suggestions about some of the special features of having twins.

General

Manual of Natural Family Planning, Anna Flynn and Melissa Brody (Allen & Unwin, 1985). Gives detailed information about natural family planning methods that will help you whether you want to become pregnant or avoid it.

Women's Rights, Anna Coote and Tess Gill (Penguin, 1974). Information guide about all aspects of women's rights. Useful for checking on maternity rights, employment, health and safety, but look for the most recent edition.

Our Bodies Ourselves, Boston Women's Collective. English edition: Angela Phillips and Jill Rakusen (Penguin, revised edition, 1985). An excellent book, covering all aspects of women's health, produced by a feminist collective. Very helpful in offering both information and support.

Let's Eat Right to Keep Fit, Adele Davis (Allen & Unwin, 1971). A direct, well-written book about healthy eating.

Miscarriage, Ann Oakley, Ann McPherson, Helen Roberts (Fontana, 1984). The first book about miscarriage with a feminist approach.

Work

How to Survive as a Working Mother, Lesley Garner (Jill Norman, 1980). Practical suggestions about organizing your life and a forewarning about some of the problems that may crop up.

But What About the Children? Judith Hann (Sphere, 1977). An analysis of childcare options for working mothers and how they operate.

Breastfeeding Guide for the Working Woman, Anne Price and Nancy Bamford (Century Publishing, 1984). An American book, adapted for British readers by the *La Lèche* League. Useful advice on how to establish breastfeeding, express milk and organize feeding around work.

Index

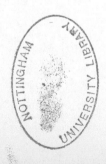